CLEAN HOUSE, CLEAN PLANET

CLEAN HOUSE, CLEAN PLANET

◆

Clean Your House for Pennies a Day, the Safe, Nontoxic Way

KAREN LOGAN

POCKET BOOKS

New York   London   Toronto   Sydney

This publication does not reflect the views of the publisher. The publication contains the opinions and ideas of its author and is designed to provide useful advice in regard to the subject matter covered. Statements made by the author regarding certain products, services, and organizations are based on the author's research and do not constitute an endorsement of any product, service, or organization by the author or publisher, each of whom specifically disclaim any responsibility for any liability, loss, or risk, personal or otherwise, which is incurred as a consequence, directly or indirectly, of the use and application of any of the contents of this book or any of the products, services, or organizations mentioned herein.

An *Original* Publication of POCKET BOOKS

POCKET BOOKS, a division of Simon & Schuster, Inc.
1230 Avenue of the Americas, New York, NY 10020

Library of Congress Cataloging-in-Publication Data

Logan, Karen.
    Clean house, clean planet : clean your house for pennies a day,
the safe, nontoxic way / Karen Logan.
        p. cm.
    Includes index.
    ISBN 0-671-53595-1
    1. House cleaning. 2. Environmental protection—Citizen
participation. I. Title.
TX324.L64   1996
648'.5—dc20
                                                96-32376
                                                  CIP

First Pocket Books trade paperback printing April 1997

10 9 8 7 6 5

POCKET and colophon are registered trademarks of Simon & Schuster, Inc.

Book illustrations by Karen Logan and Sarah Brinig
Cover design by Jeanne Lee
Front cover illustration by Pearl Beach

For information regarding special discounts for bulk purchases, please contact Simon & Schuster Special Sales at 1-800-456-6798 or business@simonandschuster.com

Printed in the U.S.A.

*It is said that the angels are drawn
to where it is clean.*

AUTHOR'S NOTE

◆

I developed a line of earth-friendly cleaners because I wanted to solve an environmental problem. I had the luxury of being able to take some time off from my computer graphics work, so for three months, I researched what I wanted to do. I decided to start by changing my own choices, habits, and purchases. As I was changing my lifestyle to be more ecological, I came across the problem of toxic products in the home. I could avoid many of them by just not buying them, but I still needed something with which to clean. The alternative cleaning products on the health-food store shelf seemed expensive and I didn't know if they would work. I found some recipes for homemade cleaners but there were hundreds of them to test. Nevertheless, they seemed easy and inexpensive. I tried out a few and was very pleased with the results, so I decided to take on the task of discovering which homemade recipes worked best.

I wanted to find the very best of the cleaning recipes that were practical and easy to make from ordinary, non-toxic ingredients. That's how this book got started. On the way, I discovered that to make using homemade cleaners practical, I needed to get "just the right kind" of bottle or container for each recipe. And to make it convenient, I needed to put each recipe right on the label. That's how my company, Life on the Planet, was born. I figured if I needed these cleaning products, so did a lot of other people out there. So . . . I sat at my desk and designed recipe labels, put them on the appropriate bottle, and called them Recipes for a Cleaner Planet.

At the time I was volunteering for the Ecology Information Center at Fred Segal's in Santa Monica, California. I met a couple of women who were starting an ecologically-oriented gift basket company called Earth Angels. They wanted to buy my cleaning products. I told them that they were hardly products yet, but they talked me into delivering some products to them nevertheless. They sold a set of them in their gift baskets for the holidays. One of the baskets was sold to a woman who gave it to her daughter for Christmas. Her daughter happened to be the actress Ally Sheedy, and my customer was Charlotte Sheedy, a well-known book agent. Ally loved my products, faxed a recipe card to her mom, and told her she thought it was a great book idea. Charlotte called me up, and we made a deal. She brought the proposal and some of my products to my wonderful editor, Emily Bestler. Emily tried the products at home and was impressed with how they really worked. She brought the book to Simon & Schuster. That's how this book got published.

In the meantime, I gave birth to my first child, a darling baby girl who has given me—along with a lot of joy—plenty of opportunities to test all of my cleaning recipes. I've continued to develop my company, Life on the Planet, which I operate out of my home, and have recipe cards, labels, and bottles with the recipes on the labels to sell. I hope you enjoy all the work and love I've put into this.

You should be aware that there may be honest differences in an evaluation of whether a cleaning product is hazardous. My view is not the only view. My evaluation of my commercial cleaning products is based on a wide variety of sources: interviews, written literature, and personal experience. I've had many interviews with company representatives, consumer-safety organizations, government agencies, Poison Control Center supervisors, hazardous-waste managers, cleaning professionals, parents, and scientists. I have tried to give you an accurate "snapshot" of what was happening with people and cleaning products in this country and not just sterile, technical descriptions. My written sources of information have come from many books, newspaper and magazine articles, material safety data sheets, government publications, and written literature from businesses. I have tried to be as accurate as possible, but you should be aware that product ingredients do change—often for the better. I am not out to prove the toxicity of commercial cleaning products, but I do want to provide generally safer alternatives. I hope I have succeeded.

Happy, healthy cleaning!

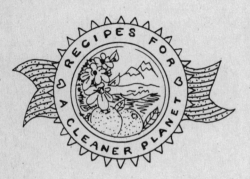

Karen Logan
Life on the Planet
(818) 880-5144

CONTENTS

PART IV

CLEANING WITH THE GOOD GUYS

PART V

THE AMAZING ALTERNATIVES

PART VI

CLEANING QUESTIONS AND ANSWERS

PART VII

THINGS TO THINK ABOUT

INTRODUCTION

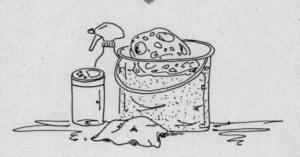

What you are about to read is a whole new approach to cleaning. These are safe, relatively nontoxic cleaners you can make at home. This book is loaded with cleaning recipes whose ingredients cost a lot less than store-bought cleaners and that really work. Nontoxic, safe, and just plain fun to use. Words like *fun* and *safe* are not usually associated with cleaning. I believe this is because, for the most part, we are used to buying and using cleaning products that are unpleasant, unhealthy, and scary to have around our children. It's no wonder that most of us *hate* cleaning. But imagine experiencing the natural scent of lemons in your nontoxic baking-soda cleanser as you finish the dinner dishes or a sweet peppermint scent as you're cleaning the bathroom floor with just vinegar and water. Imagine using great cleaners that consistently cost under a dollar. Imagine giving your young child a window cleaner that won't hurt anyone or anything *and* that really cleans. Okay, so they are more pleasant to use, you say, but do they *really* work? Yes. I have personally tested every recipe in this book and continue to be amazed by the performance of these simple combinations of nontoxic ingredients. It really is possible to make cleaning safe and more enjoyable. Read on.

P·A·R·T I

Why Switch?

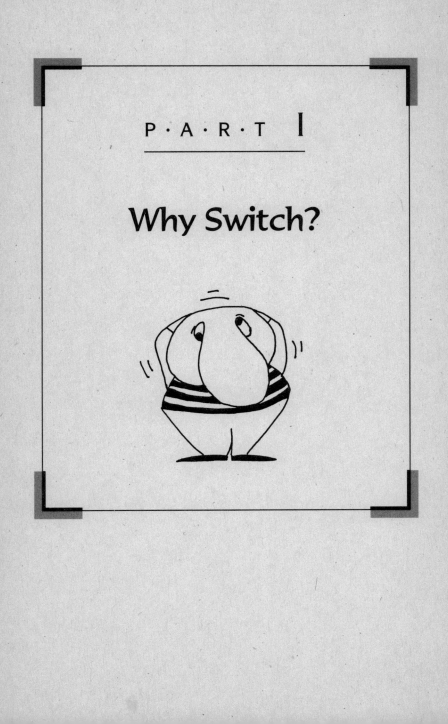

What's Really Wrong with the Chemicals with Which We Clean Today?

Here are a couple of things to think about:

- In 1989, the Environmental Protection Agency (EPA) came to the conclusion that indoor air carries a higher risk for personal exposure to toxic chemicals than outdoor air.

Where is this indoor air pollution coming from? Lots of stuff. New carpet, paint, plastics, pressboard, and natural gas. The toxic cleaning products we touch and inhale are also one of the many sources of unfriendly chemicals. No one really knows the long-term health effects of exposure to the myriad of chemicals we have brought into our homes.

- The disposal of hazardous household products is becoming an increasingly expensive problem for many municipalities.

Municipal landfills often contaminate local water and air, thus breaking federal laws that attempt to conserve our natural resources and keep our water and air clean. A landfill once labeled by the EPA as an environmentally damaging Superfund site requires expensive clean-up.

FACT: Recently, several cities in the Los Angeles area that dumped into a landfill in Monterey Park will be required to pay more than $38 million of the landfill's Superfund liability. *That settlement was based on the hazardous content of the ordinary trash from citizens that was dumped there.*

But Aren't the Chemicals in Cleaning Products Safe?

Are the chemicals in the cleaners you use safe? Maybe. Maybe not. We could set up a table of scientists who could argue about this for a very long time. Too long for me to figure out what cleaners I should and should not use.

▶ **FACT:** There are many chemicals in cleaning products that can harm you and your children.

Doesn't the Government Restrict What Chemicals Are Used in Cleaning Products?

Isn't somebody official keeping harmful chemicals out of cleaning products? *No, no, no.* Well—excuse me—that is not exactly technically correct. There is a very small list of chemicals (less than 100) that the federal government has banned because they have been determined to be too toxic to use (not just for cleaning products, but for a variety of uses). There are approximately 72,000 chemicals registered with the EPA as legal to use in cleaning products. That leaves more than 69,900 chemicals from which companies can choose.

▶ **FACT:** Complete human health and environmental effects data are available for less than 10% of registered chemicals. That means that over 90% of the registered chemicals could have some personal health or environmentally damaging effect that we don't yet know about. Our understanding of chemicals and their effects is far from complete.

Doesn't Registering Chemicals with the Government Mean They Are Safe?

No, no, no.

▶ *F A C T :* Many chemicals have been registered with the EPA based on falsified research.* Companies are often motivated by profit and not by a concern for public health. It is often too easy to just make a study say what you want it to say—and nobody can tell the difference.

What Does This Mean?

It means that companies can include very dangerous chemicals in their cleaning products and you would never know it. It can take a long time to find out and prove that a chemical is particularly dangerous and toxic to humans or the environment.

▶ *F A C T :* DDT (dichlorodiphenyltrichloroethane) was thought to be so safe when it first came out that it was even suggested that it be sprayed on the walls of children's rooms to prevent flies! Ozone-destroying chlorofluorocarbons (CFCs), the first chemicals to be internationally banned, were ironically hailed as a *nontoxic* replacement for "toxic to humans" refrigerants in the 1940s.

---

*Two major chemical testing laboratories, Industrial Bio-Test (in 1983) and Craven Labs (in 1992), have been found guilty of providing falsified research that were used to support the registration of chemicals with the EPA.

► **F A C T :** Extremely dangerous hydrofluoric acid, which can penetrate right through flesh to the bone without any warning signs of pain, is a completely legal chemical to include in a commercially sold rust remover.

Aren't Product Labels Required to Tell Us If Something Is Dangerous?

Not exactly. You don't get a complete picture from product labels. Labels will only tell you if the ingredients are poisonous, flammable, caustic, or irritating.

► **F A C T :** Labeling laws exist, but enforcement is weak. An irresponsible company's attitude can be "Who's checking, anyway?" *Many labels have unclear, misleading, and inaccurate information.* Even the safety information on some labels can be wrong!

Here's What's Not on the Label

- You won't see a complete list of ingredients on the label. *Amazingly enough, companies are* not *required to list* all *the ingredients or their concentrations on the label.* Many times, even hazardous ingredients are not listed. A poison-control manager I talked to said he would hate to have to rely on the product label alone! It also means that you, as a consumer, cannot make an educated choice about what ingredients you are willing to be exposed to. In my research for this book, I found lists of some products' ingredients and their concentrations to be quite difficult to obtain.
- You also won't see mentioned any potential long-term hazardous effect that a product might have on an individual who cleans with it regularly for years.

- Nor will you see the environmental cost and hazard of disposing of a product in sewer systems or landfills, which might one day pollute our drinking water and air. These types of hazards are completely ignored.

Are You Surprised?

Lobbying efforts by the soap and detergent industry and the Chemical Specialties Manufacturers Association are very effective. Cleaning products are big business, and spending a few million dollars to protect companies' interests is easy to do. Companies don't want to list all the ingredients because they consider them trade secrets.

▶ **FACT:** A recent bill introduced in California (Senate Bill 176) and sponsored by the Chemical Specialties Manufacturers Association would actually restrict state and local agencies from telling you about the alternatives to hazardous household products!

Doesn't the Government Protect Consumers' Interests?

The government does make efforts to protect us, but the Consumer Product Safety Commission is underfunded, understaffed, and probably overworked. They have so many products and hazards to deal with that they usually deal with only the cases involving the most deaths and injuries. They do not review cleaning products before they come on the market, and they most often respond to consumer complaints only after a product is out there.

Still Don't Believe That the Cleaning Products You Use Are That Dangerous?

Maybe the products *you use* aren't that dangerous. There are many cleaning products on the market today that *are* safe or only mildly toxic. But you should know that there are many cleaning products that are *not*. Now don't get depressed; there are alternatives.

➤ **F A C T :** Believe it or not, it takes less time to make your cleaning supplies from my recipes than it takes to buy the cleaning product from the store. Time it yourself.

◆

Do These Alternative Cleaners Really Work?

Do these homemade cleaners work? Yes and no. It's tough for safe alternative cleaners to match up to the hyperdissolving power of toxic chemicals. Nontoxic cleaners are just naturally milder. You cannot just spray these homemade cleaners on a trouble spot and watch the dirt dissolve away. That's why I have an effectiveness rating with every recipe. I want you to know ahead of time what kind of performance you can expect from each recipe. You may be pleasantly surprised. Many of these recipes work just as well or even better than their chemical competitors. Even Consumer Reports Books rated their own "homemade" cleaners at the top of their list for window cleaners and furniture polishes.

Cleaning safely requires a different kind of mindset. These recipes are the best that I could find that are safe, simple, easy to make, and effective. They do not work miracles. Some are great and some are just good enough. Nontoxic and friendly, some are even edible.*

I decided I wanted my cleaners not only to clean but to be safe for myself, my children, and the environment. Anything less is just *not good enough* for me.

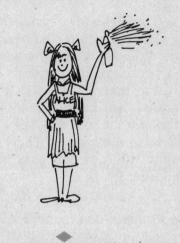

The Bottom Line

These Homemade Cleaners Are Safer for You and Your Family

Many of the chemicals in household cleaners and pesticides are not adequately tested, regulated, or controlled. *An estimated 2 to 5 million exposures to household poisons occur every year, and a significant number of them involve household cleaners.* You do not need to have these

---

*Please, use your common sense. It's a good idea not to drink or eat *any cleaner* even if it is homemade.

poisons around the house. Contact through the air or the skin and possible ingestion of these chemicals can threaten the health of you and your children.

These Homemade Cleaners Are Better for the Environment

Many household cleaning products, such as furniture polish, oven cleaners, drain cleaners, and even air fresheners, are considered hazardous waste. What's hazardous waste? It's garbage that contains chemicals that have been identified as toxic to fish, wildlife, plants, and often also to humans. You cannot responsibly throw many cleaners into the trash, but most of us do. Where does it go? Most often, to the landfill. There the toxins can leak into our groundwater, or they may pollute local streams and harm wildlife.

Using These Homemade Cleaners Will Save You Money

You probably don't realize how much money you spend on cleaners now. Because they are essential to you, you throw them into the shopping cart and you're off to the register. If you added up the cost of all your cleaners, you might be surprised how only a handful of them can add up to $20 or $30 in just a single shopping trip. It's particularly expensive if you indulge in the more toxic cleaning products like oven cleaners and pads, furniture polishes, drain cleaners, and house and garden insect sprays.

When you use the homemade alternatives found in this book, you can save hundreds of dollars. For example, on a typical visit to the store, you might purchase $20 worth of commercial cleaning products. Using an equivalent amount of homemade cleaners would probably cost you about $4.50. *If you used all the recipes in this book just* once *you would save almost $100.* Over many years, the use of safe and friendly cleaners may result in significant savings.

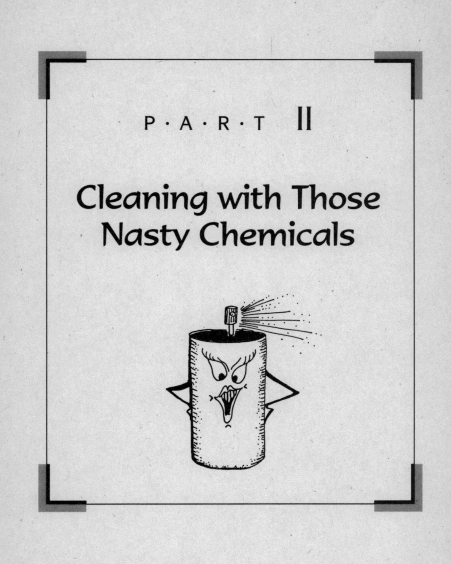

P·A·R·T **II**

Cleaning with Those Nasty Chemicals

The Bad Guys: The Truth About Those Common Chemical Criminals

Toxic chemicals are lurking everywhere in your house. Find them and get rid of them. In this section, you will find out what's potentially really bad about the chemicals in the cleaning products you buy. There are so many harmful chemicals in those cleaners that I don't have room to list them all here. I've simplified the picture and just discuss the most common chemical criminals. Don't expect to understand completely the complex world of chemicals in cleaners. Very few people do.

In what follows, I have usually described the effect of harmful chemicals as if you came into contact with them in their most concentrated form. You will probably not be affected so dramatically by exposure to a certain chemical through a cleaning product, although there are exceptions. Some cleaning products have higher concentrations of particular chemicals and therefore carry more of the hazardous chemical effect. A good example is drain cleaner, which can be almost 100% pure lye. In this case, the description of lye's damaging effects accurately represents the hazardous effect of the cleaner. On the other hand, although formaldehyde may be an ingredient in a product you use, there is usually so little of it in a cleaner that you would therefore encounter a small degree of the hazardous effect. But amounts of a chemical and concentrations can be deceiving, too. As in the case of phenol, a very small amount of it can still be quite toxic; even a 1% or 2% concentration of it can produce some hazardous effect. My descriptions that follow are meant to give you a general idea of the qualities and health hazards of a particular chemical.* I consider all of these chemicals—regardless of their range of ill effects—as potentially hazardous to my health and the environment and therefore unnecessary. You will have to determine where your safety priorities lie.

That Nasty Chemical Doesn't Just Stay in the Bottle

It's important to realize that the effect of a chemical does not stay isolated to the bottle.

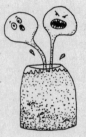

---

*The information that follows was derived from a combination of several technical references and reviewed by professionals in the field:

Gosselin, Robert E., M.D., Ph.D., Roger P. Smith, Ph.D., and Harold C. Hodge, Ph.D., D.Sc., with Jeanette E. Braddock. *Clinical Toxicology of Commercial Products.* 5th ed. Baltimore: Williams & Wilkins, 1984.

Guide to Hazardous Products Around the Home: A Personal Action Manual for Protecting Your Health and Environment. Springfield, Missouri: Household Hazardous Waste Project, 1989.

Winter, Ruth. *A Consumer's Dictionary of Household Yard and Office Chemicals.* New York: Crown Publishers, Inc., 1992.

Harte, John, Cheryl Holdren, Richard Schneider, and Christine Shirley. *Toxics A to Z: A Guide to Everyday Pollution Hazards.* Berkeley: University of California Press, 1991.

Lewis, Grace Ross. *1,001 Chemicals in Everyday Products.* New York: Van Nostrand Reinhold, 1994.

Steinman, David, and Samuel S. Epstein, M.D. *The Safe Shopper's Bible: A Consumer's Guide to Nontoxic Household Products, Cosmetics, and Food.* New York: Macmillan, 1995.

1. **When the product is manufactured,** there are many possible hazards: workers being exposed, the transportation of concentrated chemical ingredients through populated areas, and chemical waste products released into the air, land, or water.
2. **When you use the product,** you may underestimate the amount of chemical you expose yourself to. Did you realize that when you breathe, some chemicals can be rapidly absorbed into your bloodstream? Most of us don't think of it that way. We also don't realize what a sponge our skin is.
3. **When you use up the product or throw the bottle away,** those chemicals go into our environment one way or another through wastewater, garbage, or storm drains.

It's a complicated science to determine the toxicity of all of these modes of exposure, and much is still unknown. That's why keeping to simple, safe ingredients is a very smart choice for everybody.

The Bad Guys

Alcohol	Lye
Ammonia	Naphthalene
Bleach	PDCBs
Butyl cellosolve	(paradichlorobenzenes)
Cresol	Perchloroethylene
Dye	Petroleum distillates
Ethanol	Phenol
Formaldehyde	Phosphoric acid
Glycols	Propellants
Hydrochloric acid	Sulfuric acid
Hydrofluoric acid	TCE (trichloroethylene)

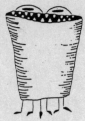

Alcohol

Found in all-purpose cleaners, disinfectants, glass cleaners, metal polishes, and more.

There are many kinds of alcohols. I've listed below the few most commonly found in household cleaners.

ETHANOL

(See Ethanol on p. 21.)

ISOPROPANOL OR ISOPROPYL ALCOHOL

Isopropanol and isopropyl alcohol are made from petroleum. When swallowed, even an ounce of them can be fatal to a small child. They act as potent central nervous system depressants. Ingestion or inhalation of them in large amounts can cause headaches, dizziness, depression, nausea, vomiting, and even coma. Those whose jobs expose them to high concentrations of alcohol have a higher incidence of sinus and throat cancers.

METHANOL

Found in windshield-washing fluids, inks, paint removers, cements, and varnishes.

Ingestion of methanol can cause inebriation, blurred vision, headache, stomach pain, weakness, blindness, and death.

Ammonia

Found in glass cleaners, all-purpose cleaners, disinfectants, floor cleaners, furniture polishes, and metal polishes. Often used as a drain cleaner, kitchen cleanser, oven cleaner, and toilet bowl cleaner.

Ammonia can be very irritating to your eyes, nose, and lungs. It can cause rashes, redness, and even burns. When inhaled in concentrated form, it can do damage to the lungs. It is dangerous in the household as a poison or when mixed with bleach to form toxic chloramine gas.

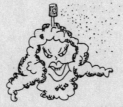

Bleach (Chlorine Bleach or Sodium Hypochlorite)

Found in cleansers, disinfectants, laundry bleaches, toilet bowl cleaners, tub and tile cleaners, and more.

Bleach is found in almost everyone's laundry room. Bleach was involved in the most frequently reported exposure noted by Poison Control Centers in the United States in 1994. When mixed with acids, bleach can form toxic chlorine gas. When mixed with ammonia, it can form toxic chloramine gas. Bleach can irritate the skin and, when ingested, the mouth, esophagus (food pipe), and stomach.

Butyl Cellosolve (in the Glycol Ether Family)

Found in heavy-duty all-purpose cleaners and degreasers, window cleaners, and more.

When absorbed into the bloodstream, butyl cellosolve can do damage to your blood, liver, and central nervous system, and can cause kidney failure. It is potentially dangerous as a cleaner because it is easily absorbed through the skin. It's best to limit your exposure until more is known about this chemical's toxicity.

Cresol (Related to Phenols)

Still found in some disinfectants, herbicides, and detergents, although many companies have phased out this chemical now because of its notable toxicity.

Cresol is a colorless, highly caustic chemical with a sweet odor. If it comes in contact with your skin, it can cause a prickly or intense burning sensation followed by the loss of feeling. Symptoms of chronic poisoning are vomiting, diarrhea, loss of appetite, headaches, fatigue, and dizziness. It is a frequent source of allergic reactions, particularly skin rashes. Exposure can cause depression, irritability, and hyperactivity and may damage the liver, kidneys, and lungs.

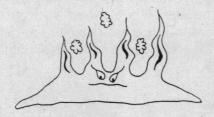

Ethanol (an Alcohol)

Found in air fresheners, disinfectants, degreasers, and metal polishes.

Ethanol is used most commonly as an antiseptic. It is clear and colorless, and, as is any alcohol, very flammable. Ingestion in large amounts can cause nausea, vomiting, coma, and death.

Formaldehyde

Found in disinfectants, furniture polishes, detergents, and water softeners. A common air pollutant emitted from particleboard, pressboard, plywood, paneling, shelves, permanent pressed sheets, mattresses, foam, plastics, and insulation. A very small amount is used in many products as a simple preservative.

Formaldehyde is a suspected human carcinogen and a common indoor and outdoor air pollutant. When exposed to higher concentrations in the air, you can develop nasal stuffiness and itchiness, red and teary eyes, nausea, headache, or fatigue. Ingestion of concentrated formaldehyde can cause stomach pain, bleeding, coma, and even death.

Glycols

Found in paints, dyes, degreasers, dry-cleaning chemicals, and floor cleaners.

Glycols can range from relatively nontoxic to extremely toxic. Many irritate the skin, eyes, nose, and throat. Exposure can cause fatigue, nausea, and tremors and can damage the kidney, liver, and central nervous system. Some glycols are harmful to the reproductive system. They can evaporate into the air you breathe, and through your lungs, they are then absorbed into the bloodstream. They can also be absorbed quickly through the skin.

Hydrochloric and Phosphoric Acids

Found in toilet bowl cleaners, metal polishes, tub and tile cleaners, and lime removers.

These potent acids can dissolve and destroy your tender tissues if you come into direct contact with them. Eyes, nose, and throat are all easily irritated by their vapors. When exposed to these acids, some people feel wheezy, sneezy, or even suffocated by them. Spills and splashes can result in burns, permanent scarring, and even blindness.

Hydrofluoric Acid

Found in rust removers and aluminum cleaners.

Hydrofluoric acid will penetrate your skin and tissue—it often doesn't stop until it reaches the bone. This type of acid is particularly dangerous because it causes no warning signs of pain.

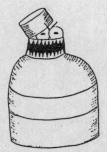

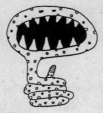

Lye (Sodium Hydroxide)

Found in tub and tile cleaners, toilet bowl cleaners, oven cleaners, and drain cleaners.

Corrosive and alkaline, when swallowed, lye will quickly eat right through your skin, face, and food pipe. When mixed with acids, lye can release harmful vapors. If it is accidentally splashed in the eyes, it can even cause blindness. It's definitely poisonous; even one drop of it in liquid or crystal form is hazardous.

Naphthalene

Found in air fresheners, carpet cleaners, mothballs, and toilet bowl cleaners.

In a concentrated form, naphthalene is dangerous to breathe and can cause headaches, nausea, vomiting, confusion, excessive sweating, and urinary irritation. It is a suspected carcinogen and is particularly toxic to small children and infants.

Serious cases of toxic exposure have resulted from infants' being dressed in clothing exposed to mothballs. It is not found in newly purchased products much anymore, as the chemical PDCB (paradichlorobenzene) has been substituted for most uses instead.

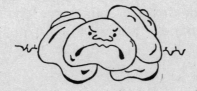

PDCBs (Paradichlorobenzenes)

Found in toilet fresheners, mothballs, room deodorants, and insecticides.

PDCBs are a white solid crystal with a wet, oily surface. They are toxic to inhale or ingest and are especially irritating to the eyes and nose. PDCBs are also used as an industrial-strength odor controller.

Perchloroethylene

Found in dry-cleaning fluid and spot removers.

Perchloroethylene is a proven animal carcinogen and suspected human carcinogen. It is a common air pollutant in dry-cleaning shops. It can cause light-headedness, dizziness, loss of appetite, nausea, and tremors, and exposure to it over a long period of time can damage the liver and central nervous system.

Petroleum Distillates (Hydrocarbons)

Found in furniture polishes, metal polishes, oven cleaners, and pesticides.

All hydrocarbons are distilled from their powerful polluting daddy, petroleum. Slippery when swallowed, these distillates can get into your lungs, causing chemical pneumonia. Ingestion in large amounts can even be fatal. Some petroleum distillates, such as petroleum jelly, are generally considered nontoxic. Others, such as toluene, xylene, benzene, and naphthalene, are considered quite toxic. Petroleum distillates can irritate the skin and can temporarily desensitize your nerve endings. They can have a pleasant odor, so watch out!

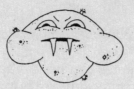

Phenol (Carbolic Acid)

Still found in air fresheners, disinfectants, and furniture polishes, although many companies have now substituted less toxic phenol derivatives.

A suspected carcinogen, phenol can cause your skin to swell, burn, peel, or break out in hives or pimples. Swallowing it may result in convulsions, cold sweats, coma, or even death. Usually only a very small amount of it is present in a cleaning product, but even a 2% solution can cause gangrene, burning, and numbness.

Propellants (Commonly Propane, Butane, and Occasionally CFCs)

Found in any aerosol product, including air fresheners, furniture polishes, and insecticides.

Propellants are easily breathed into the lungs and absorbed into the bloodstream. They are generally harmless to the skin but can be dangerous when inhaled. They are irritating to the lungs, and, in very high concentrations, they can cause irregular heartbeats. Deaths have resulted from teenagers' sniffing propellants. The average American household has 45 aerosol cans.

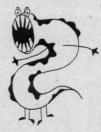

Sulfuric Acid

Found in toilet bowl cleaners and metal polishes.

Sulfuric acid fumes can be very harmful. On contact, the acid can produce severe skin burns. Even diluted, sulfuric acid can burn and scar the skin, face, and hands. Especially dangerous when splashed in the eyes, it can even cause blindness.

TCE (Trichloroethylene)

Found in spot removers and metal polishes.

TCE is a carcinogen and a narcotic! When inhaled, it can cause dizziness and sleepiness and even some memory loss. It is very irritating to the eyes and nose. On the skin, it can dissolve skin oils and cause a dry, flaky skin rash. When ingested in large quantities it can cause vomiting, nausea, and even death.

◆

Oh, the Damage Those Chemical Cleaners Can Do!

Those nasty chemicals damage more than just the environment and your health. They can damage your furniture, your floors, your carpeting, your tub, your tile, your toilets, and your pipes. So, watch out.

Do You Want Ugly Chemical Stains on Bathroom Sinks, Showers, Tubs, Carpets, and Tiles?

Toilet bowl and tub and tile cleaners can be so acidic that they can stain and pit your sinks, counters, and bathroom chrome. I've seen carpets turned green, shower stalls bleached and permanently discolored, and tubs and sinks roughened, pitted, and stained by assorted acids and cleaners. Don't use them. When you are trying to remove those stains, you could be removing the color or some of the surface you are cleaning, too! Take it easy. Commercials have trained us to think that we can just pour it or spray it on and the stain will disappear. Wrong. Only very harsh chemicals can bring about such magic disappearing acts, and they are often too harsh for me and you to use safely.

Oh, the Housekeeper Did It!

Chemical cleaners are often used by paid housekeepers, who may have little training in the hazards associated with or even the proper use of cleaner products. Some may not even be able to read the labels. Many housekeepers I know don't read English. Labels are ineffective in this situation. I've seen many a home owner point to a permanent stain and say, "The housekeeper didn't know and put this on that and ruined it." Why risk ruining expensive items such as carpet, furniture, and appliances?

Chemical Stains

Many of the products you can pull out of your cupboard and call cleaners can stain, destroy, and permanently damage clothes, furniture, and carpeting. *Chemical stains almost never come out!* I call them "positively permanent damage." Does it say that on the bottle? No.

Bleach Spots on the Carpet

I talked to my neighbor, who was using straight chlorine bleach to clean her toilet: her toddler picked up the toilet brush and dashed away. Now, her lovely blue carpet has little white spots from the bleach her toddler trailed behind. I have a feeling she's not the only one to whom this sort of thing has happened.

Wood Floors Stained and Finishes Dulled and Removed

Wood floors are particularly susceptible to chemical damage. Many all-purpose cleaners are much too strong to use on wood floors and finishes. Unfortunately, thousands of people don't know that and they go ahead and use them anyway and ruin their wood floors. Once a floor is properly finished, you rarely need anything stronger than a little bit of soap or vinegar to clean it.

Pulverized Pipes

If you talk to a plumber, he or she will tell you that liquid drain cleaners are often more effective at damaging pipes, plumbing, and people than they are at clearing drains. Don't use them!

Ohhh, My Ring . . . What Happened?

Harsh chemical cleaners are notorious for ruining precious jewelry. Pearls and opals are particularly sensitive to ordinary kitchen abrasives and other chemicals. It's better to be safe by taking those pretty items off before you clean!

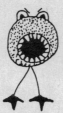

Removers Often Remove Things You Don't Want Them To.

Rust removers can put holes and pits in the top of your washer, your porcelain sinks, and glass. Often containing much too dangerous chemicals for home use, they can hurt your fingers, too!

Preventable Poisonings

It's shocking to find out that over the years, people have decided to use items like drain cleaners, toilet bowl cleaners, and rust removers to commit suicide. And toddlers can be accidentally poisoned by these cleaners if they get hold of them. Everybody knows these cleaners are dangerous. Why risk having them around the house?

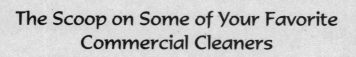

The Scoop on Some of Your Favorite Commercial Cleaners

Why shouldn't you use the stuff you have been using all these years? I can tell you why *I* wouldn't use them; then you can decide for yourself.

Pine Sol

Twenty percent pine oil is too strong for me. I find the smell irritating. And what would happen if my daughter swallowed it? When I asked the local Poison Control Center, the response was that the pine oil can be aspirated into the child's lungs and cause breathing problems, possibly chemical pneumonia. Pine oil is slippery, like gasoline, so if a child were to swallow it, it could easily slip into the breathing passage and lungs. Pine Sol also has alcohol in it. If enough alcohol is swallowed, there is no antidote, so you just have to wait and see if the child recovers. That was enough information for me. If you do use it, *please* keep it in a safe place. When I want a clean, medicinal smell, I put a little bit of tea tree oil in my homemade cleaners instead.

Tilex or X-14

I asked my cleaning-lady friends, "What's the worst cleaner that you use?" They always gave the same answer: "Tilex—it smells terrible." Reported reactions from those who use it vary from coughing, stuffy noses, and sore throats to dizziness, headaches, and nausea after cleaning a shower stall with Tilex. What's really in it? Bleach and lye or washing soap. If enough is inhaled, it can be corrosive to your lungs. You get the uglies off, but what have you done to your lungs? Don't breathe it.

Endust

Pay $4.39 for a little bit of oil and static clingy chemicals? Never. Besides, aerosol cans are expensive and the propellants in them can contribute to low-level smog. You pay a high price for very little cleaner dispensed in a fancy way.

Raid or Black Flag Ant and Roach Killers

I avoid all pesticides like the plague. I know chemically sensitive people who can walk into a room and tell me right away if it has been sprayed with a pesticide in the last 24 hours. Lethargy, teary eyes, runny noses, migraines, nausea, and the flulike aches can all be symptoms of pesticide exposure. Spray my house with a neurotoxin? I say no way.

Spray 'n Wash Stain Stick

Good news. Spray 'n Wash is a commercial product I do use! Recommended by the *Safe Shopper's Bible** as only a mild risk as an irritant. Nothing to inhale in the stick version, and easy to keep out of the reach of children. It works great.

Old English Red Furniture Polish

There's no debate here: thin, oily-type furniture polish is one of the most dangerous things to have in the house if you have a child under 6. With its inviting red fruit juice look and sweet lemon smell, Old English can seem like a tasty drink to a little one. Why are furniture pol-

---

*Steinman, David, and Samuel S. Epstein, M.D. *The Safe Shopper's Bible: A Consumer's Guide to Nontoxic Household Products, Cosmetics, and Food.* New York: Macmillan, 1995.

ishes dangerous to swallow? Because some of the children who swallow the thin, oily type furniture polish will develop chemical pneumonia, which can cause scarring of the lung tissue, causing a child to have difficulty breathing for life. To me, that's too much of a risk to have it around the house. Apparently, as of 1989, Old English changed its polish to be much less hazardous. Good for them. But I'm sure that some of you still have the old kind in your cupboards, so beware.

Comet

Comet is too harsh for my hands, making them red and irritated, especially if I have a cut or two. Also, vanity wins here. I'd like to keep my hands soft and wrinkle-free. Drying detergent-based cleaners can contribute to aging skin. Comet also has bleach in it; and when it is accidentally mixed with something like Windex, watch out—you get toxic chlorine gas. I use nontoxic baking soda instead. "But," you say, "Comet takes out stains and baking soda won't!" Okay, go ahead and keep the Comet for the stain removing, but use the baking soda for everyday cleansing. In the final analysis, I love my scented baking soda because it's much more versatile and safe. I've used the baking soda at my sink for fighting flash oil fires on the stove and soothing symptoms from spider bites on my arm. The soda snuffed out the fire and brought the swelling right down on the bite. Now, that's my kind of friendly cleanser.

Bon Ami

Bon Ami is a good choice. It is a finely grated detergent and feldspar and a fairly safe, nontoxic cleanser. Keep up the good shopping—although I still prefer a scented baking soda.

Lysol Spray Disinfectant

Do I use Lysol spray? Never. The active ingredient in Lysol spray is a registered pesticide. All disinfectants are technically pesticides. Spray pesticides and ethanol around to kill germs? No way. And, if you are using it to disinfect the air, it's ineffective, too! It's not really possible to stop or prevent the spread of germs and disease in the house by spraying a disinfectant in the air. Germs are most often spread through the air and from hand to mouth. Killing them off in one small area for a few minutes does little or nothing at all to stop them. If you look carefully at the instructions on the back of the can, they tell you to spray on *surfaces*. How many people do you know who use Lysol spray that way?

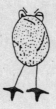

Spic and Span

Spic and Span contains phosphates, which clog up streams and rivers by encouraging the growth of algae. Although this is less of a problem today because many people buy detergents that are phosphate-free. Today, streams and rivers can get more phosphate runoff from the fertilizers we use on our lawns than they can from our detergents. Nevertheless, phosphates are things to be avoided, and responsible wastewater treatment plants try to keep their phosphate counts way down. Spic and Span now offers a nonphosphate formula. If you're hooked on this brand, get that formula instead.

Soft Scrub

Soft Scrub's a nice product. Love the way it squirts, leaves a fresh scent, and is supersoft. But it does contain bleach, which I like to avoid when I can. When products were compared in a blind test, my cleaning-lady friends unanimously chose my homemade Earth Scrub™ recipe over the commercial Soft Scrub product. Soft Scrub worked better for really dirty tubs, but for everyday use, it takes a lot of rinsing, making more work for you. And the Earth Scrub™ just feels a lot more friendly and saves you money, too!

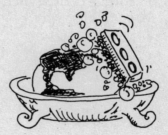

P·A·R·T III

Getting Ready to Clean Safely

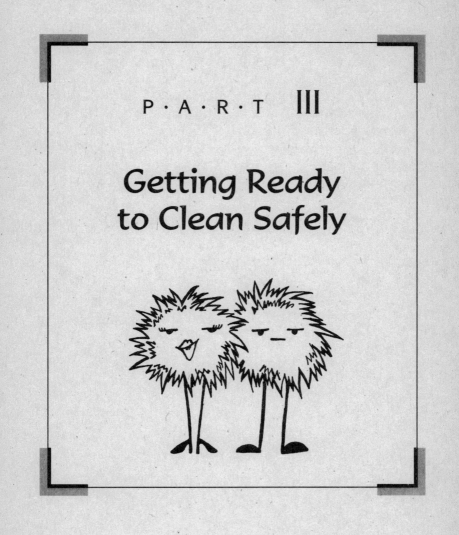

The Basic Ingredients

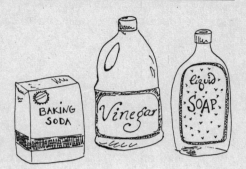

Let's get ready for a safer home.

Absolute Necessities

At a minimum, you will need some baking soda, white distilled vinegar, and some liquid soap or detergent. You'll also need several clean, empty spray-bottles, a couple of squirt-bottles, and a shaker container. You'll want some good rags and a few sponges (both white nylon and green scrubbers), and a bucket always comes in handy. Try the easiest recipes first to get started. I suggest trying the EarthShaker™ (see p. 185), Club Clean™ (see p. 156), Momma's Earth Mop™ (see p. 135), and Earth Scrub™ (see p. 239) recipes first. Once you begin cleaning with these products, it is so rewarding and enjoyable that you will want to try out more.

The Essential Oils

Good scents make cleaning fun, but you probably won't be able to get essential oils at your local grocery store. Most health-food stores carry them, or you can get them from the mail-order companies I've listed in the back of this book (see Resources, pp. 283–89). It's best to get pure essential oils, because the synthetics just aren't as good. At first I thought that the oils were a luxury, but after I tested a few of them, I absolutely loved using them.

Liquid Castile Soap

While you are at the health-food store, you will also want to pick up a bottle of liquid castile soap as a basic ingredient for many of my recipes. Liquid soaps may seem expensive, but when properly diluted, they will save you money.

Containers

You'll also need the right kind of containers. I've made a list for you to get started (see Equipment List, pp. 42–45). When using your own containers, be sure to label them properly! You don't want anyone to mistake a homemade cleaner for something else, such as a food item. You can also buy already labeled containers from my company.

Ready to Start?

Once you have all the basic ingredients, you're ready to start. Invite a friend over and make up batches of your new cleaners together. Most of the ingredients are so safe that you can even get your kids involved. You'll have fun experimenting with the fragrances. Make up several gallons of scented vinegars and three or four boxes of scented baking sodas. The first time you run out of your homemade cleaners, you may find it hard to break the habit of using another store-bought product. Head this danger off from the start. Make up several bottles while you are motivated. I usually make up three bottles of a frequently used recipe at a time. The recipes are easy to make, but in the rush of an ordinary day, it can seem hard to refill even the simplest of the recipes. Refilling is easy, if—and only if—you have all items ready and handy. I keep my essential oils in the kitchen cabinet with the spices. I keep several boxes of scented baking soda under the kitchen and bathroom sinks, and a couple of gallons of scented vinegar under one of the bathroom sinks and in the laundry room. My liquid soaps stay under the bathroom sink nearest to the kitchen. That's it. Now, let's go shopping.

◆

Shopping List

You can find most of these items in your local grocery store: baking soda, white vinegar, lemons or limes, olive oil, and club soda.

☐ BAKING SODA: Baking soda is often sold in a bright-orange box in the baking section. Arm & Hammer is a good-quality baking soda. The generic brand is less expensive, but it can clump up more easily. *Do not confuse baking soda with washing soda.* Arm & Hammer brand carries both. Make sure to *read* the box. The 2-lb. boxes are a practical size, and I usually pick up three or four of them.

☐ WHITE VINEGAR (GALLON): Heinz vinegar is a good brand. It's made from grains and not from petroleum-derived alcohols like other vinegars. I think it smells better, too! A few gallons will get you off to a good start. Don't get the brown apple cider kind. Brown vinegar is for salad dressings, not for cleaning.

☐ LIQUID SOAP (CASTILE, VEGETABLE-OIL BASED, OR GLYCERIN): You can find this type of liquid soap in the health-food store or in the health-food section of your supermarket. Most soaps are concentrated, but don't be leery of buying a large size so that you don't run out. You *will* use it all.

☐ LEMONS, LIMES, OR RECONSTITUTED LEMON JUICE: Lemon juice usually comes in a green bottle and is found with the salad dressings.

☐ ESSENTIAL OILS: Pure essential oils are made from truly natural things such as lemons, lavender flowers, and peppermint leaves. Get some from a health-food store or from a mail-order company (see Resources, pp. 283–89). The oils add wonderful scents to your cleaning formulas and can provide potential (but not proven) antibacterial, antifungal, and insect-repellent qualities. Peppermint oil is a good choice for your first oil. It's relatively inexpensive and usually liked by everyone. You can substitute peppermint or lemon extracts, but essential oils are better.

☐ BORAX: Borax is often sold in a light-green box in the laundry detergent section. I don't use borax very much in my recipes, but you might want to have it on hand for those particular recipes.

☐ **OLIVE OIL:** You'll want some olive oil (the light kind). Since you'll be using it just for furniture, the least expensive kind is fine.

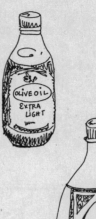

☐ **CLUB SODA:** Club soda can be found in the aisle with soft drinks or sometimes near the liquors.

☐ **PURIFIED WATER:** You'll want to pick up some purified water (or use your home purifier if you have one).

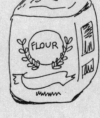

Additional Items You Should Have Around

You also might need the following items:

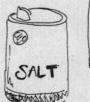

☐ Aluminum foil
☐ Vanilla extract
☐ Flour
☐ Salt
☐ Toothpaste
☐ Petroleum jelly or vegelatum (a vegetable oil–based jelly sometimes found in health-food stores)

When I approached my tightwad (and proud of it) sister about homemade cleaners, she loved the idea of making her own products and saving lots of money. "But aren't the essential oils expensive?" she asked. Yes. At first glance, essential oils do seem expensive. But remember, essential oils are the "essence" of the plant or fruit, and you need just a few drops for each cleaner. I find that a small bottle lasts me from 6 months to 1 year. At $5 to $10 a bottle per year, that's not much. And the scents add so much.

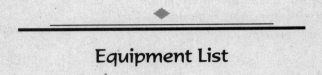

Equipment List

These are the basic pieces of equipment you will need. You probably have most of them already. Collect what you have, get what you need, and then you're ready to go.

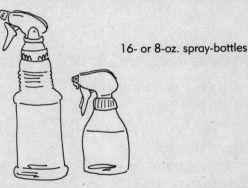

16- or 8-oz. spray-bottles

Spray-Bottles

You'll need spray-bottles of various sizes. The minimum I suggest you start with is three: one for window cleaner, one for all-purpose cleaner, and one for bathroom cleaner. Purchase as many as you can afford, up to 10. You will be using them for many things. Sounds like a lot, but it's nice to keep a few backup spray-bottles clean and prelabeled.

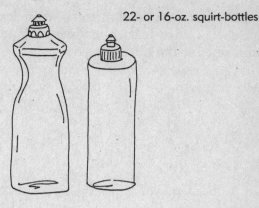

22- or 16-oz. squirt-bottles

Squirt-Bottles

I couldn't easily find any good squirt-bottles in the stores. If you are more resourceful, you might be able to find some, or you may wish to order them from my company. In a pinch, I have reused a liquid detergent bottle. If you do reuse, for safety reasons, make sure to remove or replace the label properly.

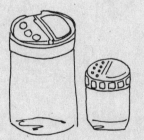

16- or 8-oz. shakers

Plastic Shaker Container with Flip-Top Lid

You'll need a shaker container with a lid and good-size holes. I bought mine in the plastic containers section of the supermarket. A good brand is the Rubbermaid Serv-in' Saver. The shaker I love to use is a reused Kraft Parmesan cheese container (the clear plastic kind with a green top, not the cardboard kind). *(Be sure to wash thoroughly and remove the old label and put on a new one. You don't want anyone to mistake your homemade cleaner for cheese!)* Get at least two shakers: one for the bathroom and one for the kitchen.

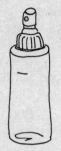

8-oz. fine-mist spray-bottle

Fine-Mist Pump Spray-Bottles

Get misters at a beauty-supply store. They're not essential, but they are nice. You will need them only for the air fresheners.

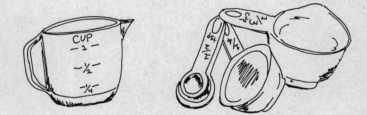

Measuring Cups and Spoons

My favorite measuring item is a large 2-cup glass measuring cup with a good pouring spout. I often mix up my cleaners right in the cup and then pour them into the container. For smaller measuring, I use a standard set of cups and spoons for ½ cup, ¼ cup, tablespoon, and teaspoon. If you are going to measure the essential oils by the teaspoon, you will need a set of *metal* measuring spoons (the oils dissolve the plastic ones). But it's easier to measure the oils by the drop right from the bottle, so that's what I suggest.

Labels and Laminating Sheets

You'll need to label your bottles and containers. Even though my ingredients are safer and less toxic than those in most commercial products, it's still important to label what you've made. Make sure to include on every label the name of the recipe and all the ingredients (including any essential oils), and don't forget the recipe! Having the recipe on the label makes all the difference in making it easy to refill the bottle. Paper labels dissolve easily in water, so it's a good idea to laminate the label before you slap it on the bottle. I get my blank labels and laminating sheets from a discount office-supply store.

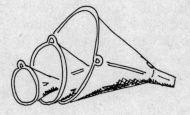

Funnels

Funnels are convenient but not necessary when filling most bottles. Even though I have quite a few funnels, I still have trouble finding mine when I need them. Pouring the mixture out of a glass measuring cup with a spout often works the best. If you do get a funnel, get the size that fits the neck of a typical spray bottle.

Getting the Best Spray-Bottles

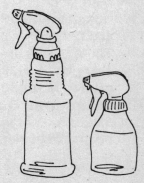

Following are some things to look for when you are getting a spray-bottle. Take a little time to get the good bottles; you'll save resources, time, and money because you will use them for years.

1. Test out the grip. Some spray-bottles are more comfortable to use than others, and this can make a difference if you are doing hours of spraying. Spray-bottles with a rounded thumb rest and a head that is angled up are easier to pump and aim.

2. Get the right size for the bottle's intended use. I use the half-size (8-oz.) sprayers for the car kit and the regular (16-oz.) for most of the spray cleaners under the sink. The larger 32-oz. sizes are generally too heavy to clean with comfortably, but I keep one or two on hand. If you have a big house or a big cleaning job, you'll want several of the larger size.

3. Try out the nozzle. Is it adjustable? Can you get both a long single squirt (good for aiming at ants) and a strong spread-out mist (for window cleaning)? Is it easy to grip and turn? Does it have an off position? You'll want an off position if you are going to give these cleaners as gifts to a friend, keep them away from your toddler, or store them sideways like in Crazy Mom's Car Cleaning Kit™ (see pp. 104–05).

4. *Look for recycled plastic content!* The best spray-bottle that I found also had the highest recycled content. Intelligence and ethics often go hand in hand. You can find the ECOLogical all-purpose sprayer (with a red cap and red house on the label) at any Target store in the hardware/cleaning section. I found mine at my local supermarket on the bottom shelf in the cleaning supplies section. You can also find the same brand but in a green-and-white-topped sprayer at any Wal Mart in the plant and garden section. These bottles are terrific and are made from 50% recycled plastic milk bottles. There is even a place on the printed bottle for a handwritten note on what you've put in them. Hurray for Sprayco, the company that makes them. I was so excited about this I called them up and managed to talk to the president. What a nice

man. Another good point is that Sprayco's bottles are assembled by physically challenged people in Michigan. All around, Sprayco is a great business to support.

5. Get more spray-bottles than you think you will need. If you think you need four bottles (two for under each bathroom sink), then get eight bottles. (See? You just forgot about under the kitchen sink.) Just close your eyes and do this. That's right, *get twice as many* as you think you'll need. Every spray-bottle will save you time and money. Don't be stingy. You may be back for even more!

I don't want to sound like an advertisement, but I do want you to get what you need, and I have to say that the easiest way to get started is to buy a sample container kit from me. If the price of buying these containers is discouraging at first, remember that you have been paying for throw-away packaging with the price of your cleaners all along. The fact is that usually between 30% and 80% of a cleaning product's price is the packaging cost alone. Now you won't have to throw those dollars away.

◆

The Sample Container Kit

Here's a description of the sample kit you can get from me to help you get started. *All the bottles come empty and ready for you to fill, using the recipes right on the label.*
Recipes for a Cleaner Planet Sample Kit #1 includes:

- Amazing Ant Cleaner™
- EarthShaker™ kitchen cleanser

- Club Clean™ glass cleaner
- Momma's Earth Mop™ floor cleaner
- It's A Lotsa Polish™ furniture polish

The kit includes a 4-oz. sample of almond or peppermint liquid soap and a ⅓-oz. bottle of lemon or peppermint essential oil and costs $19.99.

You can also purchase Sample Kit #2, which contains the following:

- Alice's Wonder Spray™ all-purpose household cleaner
- Merlin's Magic™ antiseptic soap spray
- Nature Made™ air deodorizer
- Go Spot Go™ stain and spot remover
- Dust To Dust™ furniture polish and dust spray
- Earth Paste™ tub and tile cleaner

To order, please call us at (818) 880-5144 or fax us at (818) 880-5417, or drop us a note in the mail at:

Life on the Planet
23852 Pacific Coast Hwy #200
Malibu, CA 90265

Life on the Planet

P·A·R·T IV

Cleaning with the
Good Guys

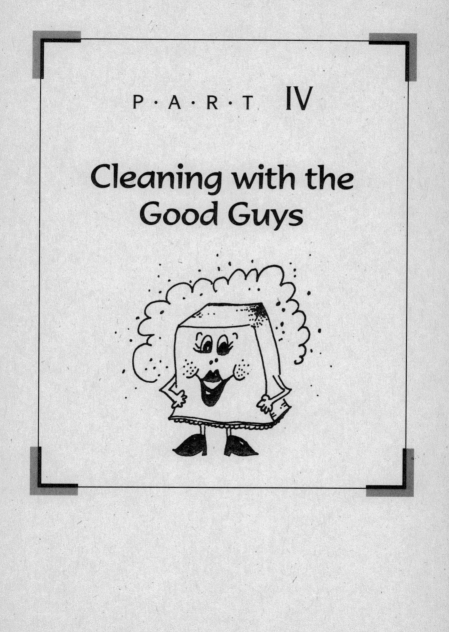

The Reasons Behind Using the Seven Basic Essentials for Cleaning

Now that you're ready, let's really get acquainted with the good guys. These basic ingredients have some remarkable qualities. Most of the recipes in this book are simply clever combinations of these seven basic ingredients.

Baking Soda (Sodium Bicarbonate)—DEODORIZER AND MILD ABRASIVE

Derived in the United States from a mineral found primarily in a 50-million-year-old dried-up lake in Wyoming, baking soda is one of the miracle natural cleansers. Not only does it absorb odors, it acts as an effective but mild abrasive in cleaning sinks, bathtubs, and counters. It is nontoxic to humans, inexpensive, and versatile.

Liquid Soap (Vegetable Oil–Based, Castile, or Glycerin)—DIRT REMOVER

Liquid soap removes dirt by dissolving the oils that bind the dirt to the objects. Soaps derived from vegetable oils are better for the environment than detergents derived from petroleum products because they biodegrade in the environment more easily and are made from less polluting ingredients.

White Distilled Vinegar (Acetic Acid, Usually in a 5% Solution)—POWERFUL DEODORIZER AND WORKS GREAT AS A CLEANING RINSE, DISSOLVING SOAP FILM AND LEFTOVER MINERAL DEPOSITS FROM EVAPORATED WATER

Vinegar is an all-purpose natural cleaner. It repels grease and grime, can help to prevent mold and mildew, dissolves soap film and mineral deposits, and even freshens the air. You can use essential oils like peppermint and lavender to soften its naturally strong scent.

Lemon (or Lime) Juice—NATURALLY ACIDIC CLEANER

Lemon juice is a powerful, natural acidic cleaner for mineral build-up, tarnish, and grease.

Salt—GREASE BUSTER, ANTIBACTERIAL, POWER CLEANER

Salt absorbs oils readily and, combined with water, can destroy any bacteria in its vicinity through a dehydrating action. The least expensive of all the homemade ingredients, it has a variety of cleaning uses, from absorbing grease to cleaning copper.

Essential Oils—FRESH, CLEAN SCENTS, AND ANTIBACTERIAL ACTION

Lemon, lavender, peppermint, and tea tree oils are all natural scents. Refreshing and even edible, food-grade lemon and peppermint oils can make great cleaning fragrances. For a powerful, superclean smell, use the popular tea tree oil, a broad-spectrum antibacterial and fungicide. (**Note:** the disinfecting power of tea tree oil has not yet been technically proven in the United States.)

Purified Water

Water, the universal solvent, is truly the most basic cleaner of all! But minerals in water can inhibit the cleaning action of any soap or detergent. Hard water makes cleaning hard. Purified or distilled water is usually soft. It's not necessary, but especially if you have hard water, it's best to use purified water for my recipes to increase their effectiveness.

◆

Home Chemistry: Lesson 1. The pH Scale

To understand cleaning you need to know just the littlest bit of chemistry. All chemicals have a pH. The pH scale ranges from acid to alkaline and is numbered from 0 to 14. Knowing the pH of a chemical can help you determine whether it's safe to use. A chemical with a pH of 7 is neutral and, if you are looking just at the pH, usually fairly safe to use. Chemicals with a pH on either end of the scale are usually dangerous because they can burn or dissolve matter. A pH of 1 is highly acidic, and a pH of 14 is highly alkaline. Soaps are generally alkaline. A mild soap has a pH of 8; a harsher soap may have a pH of 10. Drain cleaners can be as corrosive as pH 14, and toilet bowl cleaners as acidic as pH 2. But you should be aware that *pH doesn't tell the whole story.* Even though the extreme pH's are usually quite hazardous, there are exceptions. Lime juice has a pH of 1 and is quite safe to use.

Acids and alkalis tend to neutralize each other. That means that when mixed together, they tend toward a neutral pH of 7. Mixing baking soda and vinegar is a good example. Baking soda is mildly alkaline and vinegar is mildly acidic. When mixed together, they neutralize each other and form carbon dioxide gas and water at a neutral pH of 7.

Now that you know a little bit about cleaners and pH,

you can go on to learn how three of the basics—baking soda, soap, and vinegar—work together.

◆

Mixing Three of the Basics: Baking Soda, Liquid Soap, and Vinegar

Here are the rules for mixing baking soda, liquid soap, and vinegar. Pay careful attention. It's important to know how they work together.

What Happens When I Add Liquid Soap to Baking Soda?

YOU GET A GREAT CLEANER!

Soap and baking soda are both alkaline. Mixing them together makes a nice, soft, effective cleaner. Most dirt and oils are acidic. The alkaline in the soap and baking soda neutralizes the acidic dirt. That's one of the things that makes soap clean so well. Minerals in the water interfere with cleaning. Baking soda helps to soften the water and neutralizes the minerals, making the soap clean better. Baking soda also helps to lift the dirt up and away from the surface you want cleaned. Soap and soda are simple cleaners that give simply beautiful results.

What Happens When I Add Vinegar to Baking Soda?

THE BAKING SODA WILL DISSOLVE INTO CARBON DIOXIDE GAS, THE SAME GAS WE EXHALE DURING BREATHING.

Vinegar is a mild acid, and baking soda is mildly alkaline. Together, they neutralize each other in a chemical reaction that creates carbon dioxide gas and water. The carbon dioxide gas in this concentration is harmless. Try this experiment yourself. Put a little baking soda in the sink. Add a little vinegar. Hear it fizz? That's the baking soda dissolving into carbon dioxide. I use this chemical fact to clean away any baking-soda residue I might have in little corners or crevices. A scented vinegar rinse washes any residue away.

CAUTION: DON'T ADD VINEGAR TO A BAKING-SODA CLEANSER AND THEN CLOSE THE LID!

The gas from the reaction between baking soda and vinegar could make a bottle swell dangerously or break or even make the lid pop off. *If you need to soften the baking soda in a jar or bottle, please use warm* water *to dilute it instead.*

What Happens When I Add Vinegar to Liquid Soap?

CAUTION: ADDING VINEGAR DIRECTLY TO LIQUID SOAP OR DETERGENT WILL RUIN IT.

With a few of my recipes, you have to be careful about the mixing order. Don't mix the vinegar and the soap directly together. Always add the vinegar *last*. Vinegar is a mild acid and soap is mildly alkaline; therefore, they neutralize each other. That means that the vinegar dissolves the soap. I use this chemical fact by using vinegar to rinse off a soap film or residue. I love to finish my cleaning with a deodorizing vinegar rinse. Built-up soap film looks ugly and collects dirt. A fresh vinegar rinse cleans it away.

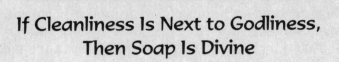

If Cleanliness Is Next to Godliness, Then Soap Is Divine

Before you start using my recipes, you should understand that there are three different types of liquid soaps.

Liquid Hand-Dishwashing Detergent

Hand-dishwashing detergent is the liquid "soap" you squirt on your dishes in the sink to wash them by hand. It's not really a soap at all, but a detergent. Liquid dishwashing detergents, such as Palmolive and Ivory, are fairly mild and good for a variety of cleaning uses. Throughout the rest of the book, I will refer to them as *liquid detergents*.

Liquid Vegetable Oil–Based Castile Soap

Liquid vegetable oil–based castile soap is a true soap. The word *castile* comes from Castilian soaps made in Italy from olive oil. Today, *castile soap* generally means a soap that is made from vegetable oils and not from animal fats. *This is the kind of liquid soap that you want to use for my recipes.* You will generally find only "real soaps" in health-food stores under brands such as Dr. Bronner's, Bio Bella, Desert Essence, and Tropical.

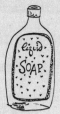

Throughout the rest of the book, I will refer to them as *liquid soaps*.

Automatic-Dishwasher Detergent

Automatic-dishwasher detergent is the stuff you squirt or pour into your automatic dishwasher. It's harsh and alkaline. You need strong stuff to make that washing automatic. *Let there be no mistake: I do not suggest the use of automatic-dishwasher detergent as an ingredient in any of my recipes.*

Note: In each of my recipes, I have told you what kind of "soap" to use, whether it's a liquid detergent or a true liquid soap. Paying attention to the difference can make a difference in the effectiveness of your cleaners.

Another Friendly Reminder

Use only *white* distilled vinegars—not the apple-cider vinegar kind—for the recipes. Apple-cider vinegar is the tasty, more expensive kind, made for use in salad dressings, not cleaning.

◆

A Note on Essential Oils

In many of my recipes, I've included essential oils. If you are chemically sensitive, you may not want to include them. Essential oils are natural but powerful chemicals and should be treated with respect. They should be kept out of the reach of children and handled with care (see my scented baking soda [pp. 247–52] and vinegar [pp. 252–55] recipes for more information on how to use them). You should be particularly carefully not to get them or put them on your skin. Spilled oils can dissolve plastics and counters, a mess that is very difficult to clean up! Even the evaporating scent can be powerful. The vapors from a pure essential lemon oil literally melted a plastic teaspoon I kept in a closed jar of scented baking soda for several months. Love them, but *respect them*. Keep your oils in a cool, dark place. Exposed to light, air, and heat, they will soon lose their wonderful fragrances.

Do Essential Oils Add Toxicity to These Cleaners?

In the amounts that I've suggested in my recipes, they don't add toxicity. A fragrance does complicate any cleaner chemically, but it can add good cleaning qualities, too, especially in the case of tea tree oil's antibacterial power. On the other hand, if you choose to use a synthetic fragrance like apple, strawberry, or peach, you could say that you are adding some toxicity to the cleaner. If you are chemically sensitive, you may find synthetic fragrances irritating, and some can even trigger asthma attacks. As with any oil, it's best not to sniff them straight from the bottle. Nevertheless, I've included a few synthetic oils in my recipes because most people love scents so much, and in such small amounts, most people won't find them to be irritating.

In general, it's best to stay with *organic essential oils* such as peppermint, lemon, lime, lavender, or tea tree. Why organic? It takes many plants to make an oil, and if the plants have been sprayed, then the oil will acquire a concentrated pesticide residue. That thought always gets me to buy organic. Oils are expensive to make, and many manufacturers mix pure oils with synthetics because it cuts their costs and it's hard to tell the difference. Check out the company you are buying oils from to make sure that they do quality tests. You want to make sure you are buying real essential oils and not fabricated mixes.

P·A·R·T V

The Amazing Alternatives

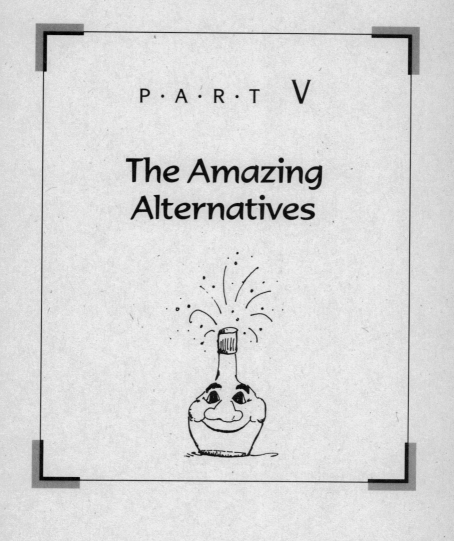

Introduction: A Note on My Ratings and Price Comparisons

Here are amazing cleaning recipes that you can live with. If I found a recipe to be a hassle to make, I threw it out. If it had some obscure ingredient that was hard to find, I tossed it. If it didn't work, you won't see it here. I've tested every one of these recipes many times over and have worked out most of the bugs in the instructions and ingredients. I use these cleaners every day and know housekeepers and other professionals who use them, too. I love them, they love them, and so will you.

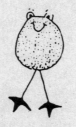

Effectiveness Ratings

I've included an effectiveness rating with most of the recipes. I've based this rating on nothing more scientific than how well I thought it should work. It's not an exact or scientific rating. It's just a general idea. First, I rated each recipe, and then I asked housekeepers, friends, and family members for their opinions. Then, I adjusted the rating. Many times my reviewers thought the recipes worked far better than I had initially rated them.

- **Effectiveness rating of 100%** means: it works great, usually better than the commercial cleaner equivalent.

- **Effectiveness rating of 80%** means: it works pretty good, does a nice job, and is pleasant and easy to use. It won't clean supertough jobs, though.
- **Effectiveness rating of 60%** means: it works but fails in some area or in some cases.
- **Effectiveness rating of 40%** means: helps to clean, but doesn't really get the job done.

Price Comparisons

The price comparisons are meant to give you a general idea of how much money you will save when you switch to a homemade cleaner. In most cases, I've picked a popular brand of cleaner at the middle of the price range in that cleaning category. All prices are supermarket retail in Southern California. You may find them to be higher than your grocery store's price. If your prices are lower, you may not save as much, but you will still save plenty!

You may notice that in each comparison, I've adjusted the amount of the homemade cleaner to match the amount of the commercial cleaner. That's why the amount of the homemade cleaner in the price comparisons will not always match the amount in the recipe. I had to adjust one amount; it was easier as I've done it.

I've tried to be detailed, fair, and honest in every comparison. Estimates on the number of uses from a commercial cleaner were based on advice from my professional cleaning friends and not on what the manufacturer claims. The price estimate for an added fragrance is the average price of several popular scents of essential oils.

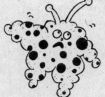

Chemical Ingredients

At the beginning of every section on a particular cleaner, I've given you an idea of what kinds of chemicals can be found in that type of cleaner. Most products contain only *some* of the ingredients listed, *not all*. I've also tried to give you a real-world description of the harm these chemicals can do. It wasn't always easy to boil down a lot of heady technical stuff into what's really harmful about a cleaner, but I've done my best.

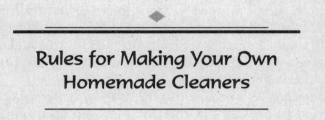

Rules for Making Your Own Homemade Cleaners

Before we start, here are some safety rules to follow when making your own cleaners:

1. *Label your cleaners properly.* Labeling can be a hassle, but if you include the recipe on the label, it will save you time later. Be sure to include all the ingredients. It's also important to label because if an accident should occur, you'll need to know what's in it.
2. *Don't reuse commercial containers.* Commercial products often do not list all the ingredients on the bottle. There may be residues of a chemical in an empty container, and you won't know what you are making.
3. *Never, ever mix commercial products. Never, ever mix commercial products with homemade products.* You don't know what you could create.
4. *Don't substitute ammonia.* I know, all you make-it-at-home types will say that you've been cleaning with

ammonia for years. But if you want to try out these recipes, please, don't call me up and tell me you used ammonia instead. I don't suggest it.

5. ***Don't use perishables like mayonnaise, ketchup, or bananas for substitute ingredients either!*** Old-time recipes that say to use mayonnaise for furniture polish or bananas to shine your shoes may seem interesting to try out, but really . . . food items like this spoil, creating bacteria and making more problems for you. *The one exception to this rule is lemon juice.* I've noted in my recipes when I think you can safely use lemon juice. Lemon juice is an effective, natural, acidic cleaner, but if left in a bottle too long, it will spoil. If I do make a cleaner with lemon juice in it, I make sure to use it all up that day or throw the rest out. But you can refrigerate it if you want to.

6. ***Basically, it's best not to try out your own mixes.*** I've tried to do this for you. Mixing even seemingly safe ingredients can sometimes yield unexpected results, so unless you know your chemistry, don't risk it.

7. ***Keep liquid soap and detergent, vinegar, and borax out of eyes!*** All of these can be quite irritating to the eyes. And don't breathe too much baking soda (breathing too much of anything particulate isn't good for you).

8. ***Please, don't eat or drink any of your cleaners.*** It's best not to get in the habit of ingesting any cleaner— toxic or nontoxic.

Air Fresheners

What's Really in Them?

Commercial air fresheners can contain a host of crazy chemicals, such as PDCBs, naphthalenes, formaldehyde, sodium bisulfate, glycol ethers, ethanol and other alcohols, assorted propellants, and synthetic fragrances.

What Harm Can They Do?

Air fresheners can be a chemical playground of gases and synthetic fragrances. Solid air fresheners can contain naphthalene, PDCBs, and sodium bisulfate, which are all quite toxic chemicals. Air-freshening sprays often contain an alcohol base with an assortment of fancy chemicals and synthetic fragrances. Allergic reactions can range from teary eyes and stuffy noses to full-scale asthma attacks. What happens when we breathe these chemicals in? Nobody really has any idea what the subtle health effects of these complicated chemical soups are. Some experts say it's wise not to inhale any of these sprays. Others would say there is too little of any one chemical in them to be of any harm. Any unnecessary suspiciously synthetic chemical is too much for me. I just don't use them. But, of course, I know all these terrific alternatives.

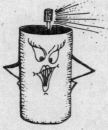

"I Love Using Aerosol Cans. Why Shouldn't I Buy Them?"

Aerosol cans have a toxic legacy. They were first used to package insecticides in the 1940s. Aerosol cans are expensive economically and environmentally. While today's

---

What's Polluting My Indoor Air?

Here are some of the many possible sources of indoor air pollution:

- New paint, carpets, plastics, vinyl, mattresses, and wood finishes
- Particleboard cabinets, pressboard shelving and furniture
- Oven cleaners, window cleaners, nail polish, shoe polish, hair spray, insecticides, typewriter fluid, and air fresheners
- Natural gas from your stove or heater
- Silicone caulking, adhesives, wallpaper glues
- Car exhaust from the garage, recently dry-cleaned clothes, marker pens, and even the ink smells from magazines and books

Put all that together in an enclosed, not always well ventilated space, and you've got indoor air pollution!

The all-time best air freshener of course is *fresh air!* Indoor air is a greater source of toxins than outdoor air.* According to EPA studies, "In all cases, personal air values exceeded outdoor air values, by ratios of two to five." Translation? Even in cities like Los Angeles, outdoor air is generally much less polluted than indoor air. So, get that fresh outside air inside. It's good for you. Often the most economical and efficient way to clean the air in your house is to just open that window and cross-ventilate. *Consumer Reports* magazine says that "just opening a few windows may do the job . . . even in winter, cracking open a window a couple of inches won't raise your heating bill by more than a few pennies an hour."

---

*Wallace, Lance A. EPA TEAM (Total Exposure Assessment Methodology) Study, Washington, D.C., Sept. 1987:2.

propellants like butane and propane don't contribute to the hole in the ozone like CFCs, they still can contribute to low-level smog. In addition, the majority of aerosol cans are thrown away to take up space in a landfill, where they sit, rusting and leaking their chemical contents into our ground, water, and air. Partially full aerosol cans can also explode in the garbage or at landfills, occasionally causing fires and injuries to disposal workers. Do I want to contribute to that possibility? No, thank you. For almost every use, pump sprays work just as well.

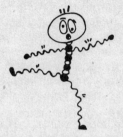

Friendly Green Toxin Eaters
Natural Air Cleaners

Most air cleaners won't even touch the majority of the chemicals and gases we consider to be toxic indoor air pollutants. To fight this influx of chemicals into our bodies, we can use our friends from nature, plants. According to a 2-year NASA study, ordinary indoor plants can be very effective at absorbing toxic indoor chemicals in the air. All plants clean and condition the air to a certain degree, but some plants are particularly good at absorbing specific chemical air pollutants. What great air cleaners! Use them. They take only a little water and love, and they give back so much in beauty and health.

- To offset the benzene from your gas stove when you are cooking or baking, keep an **English ivy** plant in your kitchen.
- To capture a variety of chemicals, including the TCE from new paint, the benzene from new plastics, and the formal-

dehyde from new cabinets or shelves, make sure to buy two or three pots of colorful **chrysanthemum flowers**. They also make great housewarming gifts.

- To absorb the formaldehyde outgassing from your press-board office or computer furniture, keep a **spider plant** or two on your desk or top shelf. Get a large, easy-to-care-for **corn plant** for the office, too, because you'll need to absorb the formaldehyde from new paper, books, cardboard, and pressboard bookshelves.
- If you just installed foam insulation or a foam carpet pad or have new foam furniture, add a few **azaleas** to your table tops.
- Eliminate the fumes from the products, oils, gasoline, and carbon monoxide in your garage by installing several **spider plants**, **English ivies**, and **dracaenas** on window sills, shelves, and in corners. Place them where they can get at least a little sunshine, and try to keep those garage doors and windows open for ventilation whenever you can.
- Indoor air pollution experts recommend one plant for every 100 feet.
- Other powerful air-filtering plants are **Chinese evergreens, golden pothos, Gerbera daisies, bamboo palms, dieffen-bachias, and peace lilies.**

Effectiveness Rating: 90%

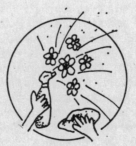

There are so many fun ways to freshen the air nontoxically. Here are a few of the best.

Nature Made™
Odor Absorber

This fine-mist spray homemade air freshener really works to absorb odors, not just cover them up. I use this one for the bathroom, but it works great for kitchen odors, too.

Ingredients: White distilled vinegar and an essential oil for fragrance—I suggest peppermint. I also like to use Heinz vinegar for this recipe because I think that brand smells better than others.

What Else You'll Need: An 8-oz. fine-mist spray-bottle. You can usually get one at a beauty-supply store, or you can buy a labeled one from me.

How to Make: Fill your spray-bottle with white distilled vinegar. Add 20–30 drops of your favorite oil. Shake before using.

How to Use: Spray to absorb unpleasant odors. Great for the bathroom and kitchen. Spray-mist an area and leave the room. *Do not put your face into the mist and sniff the spray.* Unlike commercial air fresheners, this air freshener is meant to absorb the odor and is not meant to be inhaled as a sweet smell. The odor will be gone in minutes. I make sure to have a bottle on the counter in the bathrooms whenever I have guests. I've also used Nature Made™ when changing a diaper pail or emptying out a stinky garbage can. A few squirts makes the job much more pleasant. Great for onion, cabbage, and garlic kitchen odors, too. **Caution:** Vinegar is a mild eye irritant, so be careful not to spray it in your eyes or let your kids get hold of it and spray it in theirs.

Effectiveness Rating: 90%

Commercial Brand* vs. Nature Made™ (9 oz. of spray air freshener): $1.43 vs. 48¢. A little over a cup of vinegar will cost you 18¢. Your own choice of special scents will cost 30¢ or less. You'll **save** 95¢ each time you refill the pump.

---

*Price comparison with Glade air freshener.

Good Clean Scents
Solid Air Freshener

Simply a box of scented baking soda, this subtle bathroom deodorizer is very handy as a cleaner, too. Just dip a sponge into the box and start cleaning.

Ingredients: Baking soda, a box, and an essential oil for fragrance.

What Else You'll Need: A decorative 2″ × 5″ cardboard box. (I found mine in a stationery store.)

How to Make: Put some baking soda in a pretty box. Add 5 to 10 drops or more of your favorite essential oil and mix.

How to Use: Keep the box uncovered or the lid open halfway over it. This naturally scented baking soda subtly deodorizes and helps to keep the bathroom smelling fresh and clean. Essential oils do evaporate over time, so re-scent your soda as often as you like. My favorite bathroom scent is lemon and lime. I keep a couple of boxes of scented baking soda ready under the sink for easy refills.

Effectiveness Rating as a deodorizer: 50%

Effectiveness Rating as a handy cleaner: 80%

Commercial Brand* vs. Good Clean Scents (solid air freshener): $1.77 vs. 30¢. The ½ cup of baking soda will cost you 15¢, the fragrance about 15¢. You'll **save** $1.47.

---

*Price comparison with Renuzit.

Terrific Toothpaste Reserves!

Every once in a while, I run out of toothpaste before I remember to get some more at the store. In a pinch, I use a peppermint oil–flavored baking soda as a backup toothpaste. It doesn't taste great, but it does the job. Don't use much more oil than is already in this recipe; mix well. Use only *food-grade* peppermint oil, of course.

Keep Your Drains Clean and Fresh, Too

After 2 months, the baking soda will have finished deodorizing, and you can dump it down your drains. Pour in a little vinegar, let it fizz and sit for 15 minutes, then rinse the sink thoroughly with hot water. This easy routine will help to keep your drains deodorized and running smoothly.

Vinegar is a powerful deodorizer. Here are a few recipes that show you how to take advantage of its natural power.

For That Kitchen Garbage-Pail Smell
Garbage-Can Deodorizer and Cleaner

Odors are often Nature's way of telling us that something needs cleaning. On the other hand, we don't want to clean it because it smells! Overcome that cleaning avoidance syndrome by using the deodorizing power of baking soda first to douse that smell!

Ingredients: Baking soda and an essential oil.

How to Make: Make a scented baking soda and sprinkle about ¼ cup of it into the bottom of your garbage pail.

How to Use: The first thing that I do for any smelly old thing is to dump some freshly scented baking soda on it. A bad odor will drive you away, but the baking soda makes the cleaning job *almost* pleasant. Then you can clean out the garbage can. To avoid clogging drains, rinse it outdoors if possible. Go back into the house, and wipe clean with a soapy cleaner and some hot water. Let it dry, and then sprinkle more baking soda in the bottom. The baking soda at the bottom will help keep your can dry and mildew-free as well as mildly deodorized. The soda makes a nice paste to clean with next time I rinse it out.

Effectiveness Rating: 70%

For That Smelly Garbage Disposal

Lemon Iced

Odors accumulate in disposals around the blades, underneath the rubber rims, and in the sink trap in the pipe. Grease is notorious for causing disposal problems and odors. Here's how to help you degrease it and make it smell fresh at the same time.

Ingredients: Citrus peels (any kind will do) and some ice cubes.

What to Do: Drop three or more ice cubes and a couple of fresh citrus peels down your disposal and grind them. Very noisy, but what a great smell! The ice cubes help to cool any grease and grind it out. The citrus peels add a refreshing scent and have a natural acid cleaning power.

Effectiveness Rating: 80%

How to Prevent a Smelly or Clogged Garbage Disposal

Rule #1: Don't pour grease down the disposal! Hot, un-rinsed grease will stick to every little crevice in your disposal. But if you do, rinse as soon as possible with hot, hot water. The hot water helps the grease to rinse down the drain. To pressure-clean your disposal, some manufacturers suggest you fill the sink with water and then turn on the disposal to flush.

Rule #2: Don't stuff potato peels, gobs of rice, or tons of sticky pasta down your disposal, expecting it to turn it into liquid. It won't! Silly mistakes like this keep plumbers fat and happy on your dough.

Rule #3: Compost your food scraps instead of throwing them down the drain or into the garbage. My sister and I both have bins outside where we put our food scraps. Add some worms, and you have an automatic composting machine. The worms actually eat the garbage and turn it into great garden soil. Our 2-year-olds love the worms, and we love the rich, dark soil. Many adults are repelled by worms, but it's an aversion worth getting over. Most kids love them.

Vanilla Power

Air Freshener

This is a sweet, simple, and surprisingly effective air freshener. You'll be amazed by the results.

Ingredients: A cotton ball and pure vanilla extract (not the imitation kind).

What Else You'll Need: A small jar, dish, or bowl.

How to Make: Put the cotton ball into the container and soak it thoroughly in the pure vanilla extract.

How to Use: Place the jar, uncovered, in the area you want freshened. Voilà! It starts working in even 1 hour, but after 8 hours or so, you'll smell a significant difference. The cotton ball will dry out. You can reuse it, but it works better if you add a new cotton ball instead. The vanilla adds a very pleasing odor and sops up some really bad ones. Works best in an enclosed space like closet, bathroom, or car. Keep it in a jar for the car and take the lid off at night to freshen while you sleep. It's good for smoke odors, too—it's an especially good gift for someone who doesn't like smoke but lives with someone who does. A friend of mine had an old Karmann Ghia convertible that smelled bad in the interior; after a couple of days of my cotton-ball treatment, it smelled sweet. Ah, the rewards of simple things.

Effectiveness Rating: 55%

The Orange Planet
Closet Deodorizer

I used to make these homemade air fresheners as Christmas gifts as a kid. Your kid will love making them, too!

Ingredients: An orange, a bottle of whole cloves, and a ribbon.

How to Make: Get out a fresh orange and a bottle of whole cloves. When you are watching TV or otherwise relaxing, you can entertain your hands by poking the cloves into the orange until the entire surface is covered.

How to Use: Tie a ribbon around it, and hang in a closet or any area you need deodorized. Makes a great holiday gift.

Effectiveness Rating: 60%

Plastic Odors Be Gone
Odor Absorber

Plastics can absorb some unpleasant odors that are hard to get rid of. Soak them in vinegar, and the odor is gone.

Ingredients: A scented vinegar.

How to Make: See scented vinegar recipes on pp. 252–55. For this recipe, I like to use the powerful tea tree oil for that superclean smell.

How to Use: After 1 1/2 years of use, my plastic diaper pail had absorbed lots of icky odors. No matter how many times I washed and rinsed the pail, the odor still remained. What to do? I dumped some scented vinegar in the bottom of the pail, swished it around, and let it sit for a couple of hours. I rinsed the pail out and voilà, the odor was gone. No commercial product I've found can match that vinegar power. Use this trick for your plastic garbage cans as well. If you are watching your pennies, you can probably use a lot less vinegar.

Effectiveness Rating: 100%

Vinegar Mop
Air Freshener

This air freshener is reputed to clean up even skunk odors. I've never tried it for that—I hope I never will!

Ingredients: White distilled vinegar.

What Else You'll Need: A small bowl or jar.

How to Make: Put about ½ cup of vinegar uncovered in a bowl or jar.

How to Use: I usually place this on an upper shelf and let it sop up the odors. This is assuming that you don't continue to create the smell at a faster rate than the vinegar can take it away, which certainly can be the case if you let your kitchen garbage can continue to ripen and expect the vinegar to do the job. This trick is also good for mopping up some offensive cooking odors, musty closet smells, smoky rooms, or kitchens with little or no ventilation.

Effectiveness Rating: 40%

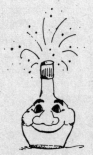

Bowl You Over

Toilet Bowl Deodorizer

Do you try to save water by not flushing the toilet? Then you really need this recipe.

Ingredients: White distilled vinegar and an essential oil.

How to Make: Make a scented vinegar according to my scented vinegar recipes (see pp. 252–55).

What to Do: To deodorize the toilet bowl, pour 1/2 to 1 cup of scented vinegar into it. If you are brave enough to put your nose near the bowl, you can instantly smell the difference. The vinegar actually helps to break down the uric acid. Now, you can save water all day without having to worry about an odor.

Effectiveness Rating: 100%

Last but not least, our pets cause odors, especially indoors. Kitty litter boxes can be particularly smelly. Here's an inexpensive and effective remedy.

Casey Kitty's Litter Box Deodorizer

Casey the Kitty is my daughter Sophie's favorite cat; she belongs to our neighbor, Laurie. We can't have cats because Sophie's daddy is allergic to them. Casey is a most friendly cat and willingly endures the normal toddler abuse, tail-pulling, squishing, stepping, eye-poking, and squeeze-hugging from my daughter. She almost seems to enjoy it. Casey, of course, has a litter box. Here is how her litter box is freshened. Casey loves it. She likes the eucalyptus and peppermint scents the best.

Ingredients: Baking soda and an essential oil for fragrance (I suggest eucalyptus, peppermint, or lavender).

How to Make: Scent approximately 2 cups of baking soda (about half of a regular 2-lb. box) with any *one* of the following oils: 24 drops of eucalyptus oil, 24 drops of peppermint oil, or 20 drops of lavender oil.

How to Use: Pull open the entire top of a 2-lb. baking soda box. Add the essential oil on top of the baking soda (right in the box) and mix it in with a fork. Pour in about 1 cup of the scented baking soda into the bottom of the litter box. Add the sand last. Save the rest of the baking soda for the next time.

Casey Kitty's Litter Box Deodorizer has a lot of advantages over the store-bought product. First of all, it costs a lot less. Second, you can choose any scent you like. Third, if you keep the box in a closet or small, enclosed room, you will find the area delightfully scented by the fragrance. Over time, your plastic litter box will absorb some of the oil's scent and smell fresh rather than dirty. The baking soda at the bottom of the litter box also makes it easier to clean.

Effectiveness Rating: 95%

Commercial Brand* vs. Casey Kitty's Litter Box Deodorizer (20-oz. cat litter box deodorizer): $2.44 vs. 99¢. The 2½ cups of baking soda will cost you only 75¢. The fragrance costs about 24¢. You'll **save** $1.45.

---

*Price comparison with Arm & Hammer cat litter box deodorizer.

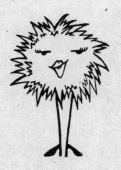

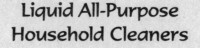

Liquid All-Purpose Household Cleaners

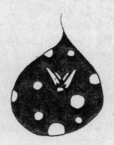

What's Really in Them?

Typical ingredients in liquid all-purpose cleaners include ammonia, alcohol, bleach, butyl cellosolve and other glycols, detergents, dyes, fragrances, and sometimes fine plastic particles.

What Harm Can They Do?

Many all-purpose cleaners on the shelves today are much too strong for ordinary household use. Most try to do too much, too quickly. The soapy ones are difficult to rinse and leave floors sticky. The smelly ones are so strong that they can irritate sensitive lungs and noses, corrode metal, and are even poisonous. If you use this type of cleaner straight from the bottle, it can damage paint, metals, and other sensitive surfaces. Other all-purpose cleaners contain ammonia, which is irritating to breathe and dangerous when mixed with bleach. Almost all contain unnecessary and potentially irritating dyes and fragrances.

Many all-purpose cleaners used by professionals contain the chemical butyl cellosolve, which can be absorbed very quickly through the skin and into the bloodstream. In high concentrations, butyl cellosolve is known to do damage to the kidneys and liver. Companies that sell products with butyl cellosolve in them will argue there is not enough in the product to do you harm. On the other hand, I know of at least two well-respected cleaning professionals who avoid cleaning products containing *any* butyl cellosolve at all.

Don't get me wrong—some of the all-purpose cleaners on the shelf are safe and relatively mild to use. The environmentally conscious Washington Toxics Coalition's *Buy Smart, Buy Safe* guide lists these, among others, as generally acceptable alternatives: Planet concentrated all-purpose liquid, Ajax lemon fresh liquid, Mr. Clean liquid (nonphosphate), and Spic and Span liquid (nonphosphate). Simple castile soaps, like Dr. Bronner's, rate at the top of their list as the very lowest in toxicity and environmental impact. For all-purpose cleaning, I use either a liquid soap or the liquid detergent at my sink. Here are my suggestions for using both.

Dishy-Wishy Washer
All-Purpose Cleaner

Liquid hand-dishwashing detergents are excellent, often overlooked, all-purpose cleaners. Pleasant and generally mild to your hands, you'll save packaging and money by using them. The only problem I've found is that it's easy to use too much. You need only a very little to make a fine all-purpose cleaner.

Ingredients: Any liquid hand-dishwashing detergent and water. And, perhaps, some scented vinegar as a rinse.

What Else You'll Need: A spray-bottle, squirt-bottle, or bucket.

How to Make: Use 2 or 3 squirts of liquid detergent for a bucket of warm water, 1 tsp. for an 8-oz. spray-bottle of water, or 1 tbsp. for a 16-oz. squirt-bottle of water. For the vinegar rinse, use my Momma's Earth Mop™ floor cleaner recipe (see p. 135) and squirt on directly. Or for big jobs, use 1 to 2 cups of scented vinegar per bucket of rinse water.

How to Use: It's important to dilute the liquid detergent properly. Making lots of suds means making lots of work rinsing. If you do end up using too much detergent, you can remove the residue with a vinegar rinse.

- For washing floors, walls, windows, and baseboards, use the same 1 or 2 squirts per bucket of warm water. To make things come squeaky clean and smell nice, I usually follow up with a scented vinegar rinse.
- For hand-washing delicates, use a tiny squirt for a sinkful of water and rinse well.
- For presoaking stains and stain removal, use just a dab.
- For washing your car, liquid detergents are great soil and grease cutters. Use 2 or 3 squirts in a bucket of warm water.
- For most stubborn dirt or stains, letting the stained item soak in a liquid detergent solution and then scrubbing with a white nylon-backed sponge usually does the trick.

Effectiveness Rating: 95%

Commercial Brand* vs. Dishy-Wishy Washer (64-oz. all-purpose cleaner): $4.35 vs. 35¢. The liquid dishwashing detergent costs less than 1¢ a squirt! About 35¢ worth of dishwashing liquid makes about 40 gallons. You'll **save** $4.00.

---

*Price comparison with Fantastik.

Baking soda is also used more and more these days as an all-purpose cleaner. Some painting companies use it as an alternative to chemical paint removers or light sandblasting. Baking soda has also proven itself indispensable as a chemical spill "neutralizer" and cleaner-upper. Those in charge of "toxic" clean-ups say they couldn't live without it.

It's also important to note that hot, hot water and

steam are naturally great cleaners. Many tough jobs like city street cleaning are handled with steam-cleaning machines and only a little detergent. Remember, boiling water is an excellent disinfectant, too.

Dr. Bronner's Sal Suds

One of the best all-purpose cleaners that you can buy off the health-food store shelves is Dr. Bronner's Sal Suds. Pine Sol lovers will like Sal Suds as a substitute because it has that lovely, familiar pine scent. Sal Suds works great on hard surfaces like the floor, walls, painted woodwork, cars, aluminum siding, and even boats.

Environmentally speaking, Sal Suds rates at the top. You can buy it in a quart-size bottle at your local health-food store or co-op. It may seem more expensive, but, diluted to the correct amount, it's less expensive than many of the brand-name all-purpose cleaners. Use it in about the same amounts as you would a liquid detergent, or perhaps a little bit more: 2 tbsp. for a bucket of warm water, 1 tsp. for an 8-oz. spray-bottle of water, or 1 tbsp. for a 16-oz. squirt-bottle of water.

One of the advantages that Sal Suds has over a brand-name liquid detergent, like Palmolive or Ivory, is that it is very easy to rinse and doesn't leave a sticky film. Easy rinsing is important because it saves work, time, and water. That puts Sal Suds on the top of my all-purpose cleaner list.

Commercial Brand* vs. Sal Suds (15-oz. all-purpose cleaner): **$1.40 vs. 90¢**. Sal Suds, used at a concentration of 1 tbsp. per gallon, costs 12¢ per gallon. At a concentration of ¼ cup per gallon, a bottle of Pine Sol makes about 7½ gallons. You'll **save** 50¢ each time you make a purchase.

*Price comparison with Pine Sol.

◆

Spray All-Purpose Household Cleaners

What's Really in Them?

The same basic ingredients in the liquid all-purpose cleaners are found in spray all-purpose cleaners, but in less concentrated form. Typical ingredients include ammonia, alcohol, bleach, butyl cellosolve and other glycols, detergents, dyes, fragrances, fine plastic particles, and lots of water.

What Harm Can They Do?

Most spray all-purpose household cleaners are fairly safe to use. Generally speaking, they are technically not very toxic because of the dilution. *But, you are paying a premium for mostly just water.* Still, I find your typical spray irritating to breathe. I just can't seem to use them without inhaling them. I get a temporary sore throat every time I use them. My 2-year-old always coughs when she is in a room where they've been sprayed.

After a lot of experimenting, I found that the best homemade alternative was a simple mixture of vinegar, borax, soap, and water. Because this recipe seems so "wonderful" and not Fantastik, I've called it Alice's Wonder Spray™.

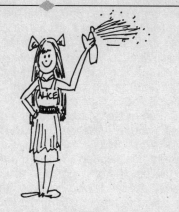

Alice's Wonder Spray™
All-Purpose Household Cleaner

This recipe has a little bit of mildly toxic borax in it. Although technically not a disinfectant, borax is reputed to have antifungal and antiseptic qualities. Borax is toxic to ingest, so please be sure to label the bottle with the ingredients, and keep out of the reach of children.

Ingredients: Liquid soap or detergent, white distilled vinegar, borax, purified water, and an essential oil for fragrance.

What Else You'll Need: A clean 16-oz. trigger spray-bottle.

How to Make: Mix 2 tbsp. of vinegar with 1 tsp. borax. Fill the rest of the bottle with very hot water. Shake until the borax is dissolved. Add the ¼ cup of liquid soap or ⅛ cup of liquid detergent *last*. To scent, add 10 to 15 drops of an essential oil. I like to use a combination of lavender and lemon. Because minerals in the water inhibit cleaning, it's best to use purified or distilled water, especially for this recipe.

It's important to dissolve the borax in hot water so that it doesn't clog the spray nozzle. And don't mix the soap and vinegar directly together, because the soap will clump up. Please, follow the order of the recipe by mixing the vinegar, borax, and water first and adding the soap last.

How to Use: Spray and wipe. Use Alice's Wonder Spray™ as you would any other all-purpose household cleaner. I use it on my refrigerator, walls, tile, shower, and toilets. It's not as chemically powerful as commercial cleaners, but if you *give it a little more time*, it works just as well. To help remove or prevent mold and mildew, use 1 tbsp. borax instead of 1 tsp.— and hotter water to make sure it dissolves. **Caution:** Borax is an eye irritant and can be harmful if swallowed. Keep this product out of the reach of children. Do not use if you have open cuts on your hands and skin.

I keep a couple of spray-bottles of Alice's Wonder Spray™ underneath both the kitchen and bathroom sinks. I use enough to have several bottles conveniently placed around the house. My husband has cleaned the white melamine furniture with it and claims that it works great. It also makes a good shower wall cleaner. A friend, who loves to clean but is plagued with allergies, said this after cleaning her shower with it: "For once, when I was cleaning I wasn't sneezing or getting stuffed up."

Use Alice's Wonder Spray™ to:

- Clean your refrigerator walls, drawers, and shelves. It works great, smells great, and helps to prevent mold.
- Remove fingerprints on walls, doors, cabinets, and drawers. If you need it, use a little sprinkle of baking soda on your rag for extra scrubbing power. The soap in Alice's Wonder Spray™ helps to clean doorknobs, too.
- Wipe down the toilet seat and around the toilet area.
- Clean and deodorize the insides of trash cans.

Effectiveness Rating: 70%–80%

Commercial Brand* vs. Alice's Wonder Spray™ (22-oz. all-purpose cleaner): $2.69 vs. 23¢. 1 tsp. borax costs about 1¢; 3 tbsp. vinegar, about 2¢; 1 tsp. good-quality soap, about 2½¢; and scent, about 10¢. To bring the amount of spray up to 22 oz., add about 5¢. You'll **save** $1.46 each time you refill the bottle.

---

*Price comparison with Formula 409.

WHAT MAKES ALICE'S WONDER SPRAY™ SO WONDERFUL?

It has no ammonia. I belong to the "I-hate-ammonia club." Ammonia is very irritating to the eyes and lungs. Children and adults with colds, asthma, bronchitis, or other respiratory problems are particularly sensitive to it. Even at low concentrations, it can be very irritating to the eyes and lungs. You increase the risk of irritation when the ammonia is sprayed into the air. Now you never need to use ammonia again.

CAN ALICE'S WONDER SPRAY™ CLEAN CRAYON AND PENCIL MARKS OFF WALLS AND DOORS?

Yes, with a little extra help from baking soda. Wet the wall with Alice's Wonder Spray™. Sprinkle a little soda on your rag and rub. Don't rub too hard, or you will remove the paint. Follow up with a good squirt and wipe of Alice's Wonder Spray™. I think that with a little bit of added baking soda power, it performs better than any other commercial brand that I've tried.

◆

Automatic-Dishwasher Detergents

What's Really in Them?

Ingredients of automatic-dishwasher detergents include phosphates (often, chlorinated trisodium phosphate), sodium carbonate (washing soda), sodium silicates, and chlorine bleach.

What Harm Can They Do?

Most automatic-dishwasher detergents contain harsh chemicals and phosphates to help them clean automatically. They can also be dangerously alkaline, with pHs ranging from 10.5 to 12. Swallowing can cause burns. Please, don't let your baby get into that open dispenser filled with detergent! Most kids who do end up with just a burn on the lip or tongue, but the detergent can burn the stomach or food pipe (esophagus) if they swallow enough of it. *Not putting* any *detergent in the open dispenser (the one without a lid on it) makes the situation much safer for those curious hands and mouths.*

I tried, but I couldn't find a homemade alternative that really worked. I still buy a commercial automatic-dishwasher detergent. Here's how I make the best of the situation.

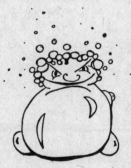

Dish Sprinkle™

Automatic-Dishwasher Detergent— the "Lazy-Day" Dishwashing Way

After a relaxing, satisfying dinner, who feels like doing the dishes? No one. This is my family's solution to cleaning up the dishes in the most lazy and effortless way. The folks at Arm & Hammer's 800 telephone number (printed on the baking-soda box) suggested this idea to me, and I modified it to make the most effortless, automatic dishwashing in your house ever.

Ingredients: Baking soda.

What Else You'll Need: A shaker (for suggestions on the type of shaker, see the information after my EarthShaker™ recipe on pp. 185–86).

How to Use: As you are piling the dirty dishes in the sink, scrape off the lumpy food and shake on some baking soda. This is a fast and easy way to cut down on odors as well as getting a start on dissolving the grease and grime. The baking soda works best if slightly wet. Use more for the stuck-on food and greasy dishes. Let the wet baking soda sit on the dishes for a least 5 minutes. *You've started your automatic dishwashing the minute the soda touches those dishes.*

Here's the lazy-day part. You don't have to load the dishes right away. Yes, you can leave them in the sink for hours, even days! The damp baking soda will keep them sweet-smelling and the food soft. Use a spray-bottle of water to dampen them if you like. Now, when you're feeling a bit more energetic, you can load those dishes from the sink straight into the dishwasher. *No rinsing required.* Add your dishwashing detergent *to the closed dispenser only* and start the machine. Glistening, gleaming dishes will await you. This simple procedure absolutely eliminates the need to put extra automatic-dishwasher detergent in the open dispenser. You can reduce the amount of detergent you use in the closed dispenser as well. Try just filling it up only halfway. You'll be amazed at how little you can use.

Here's the price savings: Let's say that right now you are using 5 tbsp. of commercial detergent in your dishwasher: 3 in the closed dispenser and 2 in the open dispenser. Right away, you can eliminate 2 tbsp. in the open dispenser, and you should be able to cut down by at least 1 tbsp. in the closed. *Your automatic-dishwasher detergent bottle will now last twice as long.* That's half as expensive, right? Not quite. Don't forget, you have to add in the extra cost of the baking soda. Practically speaking, I use the baking soda on only the dirtiest dishes and only some of the time. I've still been able to reduce the amount of automatic-dishwasher detergent I use by one-fourth. Now, that's a real price savings.

Effectiveness Rating: 100%

Commercial Brand* vs. Dish Sprinkle™ (50-oz. automatic-dishwasher detergent): $3.17 vs. $2.37. If you use about ¼ cup of baking soda for each load, it will cost you about 8¢. You will probably save 10¢ worth, or 3 tbsp., of detergent each load. You reduce the amount of phosphates, packaging, and water consumed and save a little money, too. If you use a little bit more than ¼ cup of baking soda each time, you'll probably **break even**.

*Price comparison with Cascade Lemon Liqui Gel.

Be Stingy with That Automatic-Dishwasher Detergent

The detergent receptacles in your dishwasher allow you to easily exceed the amount of dishwashing detergent you really need. The closed dispenser cup on most dishwashers accommodates more than 3 tbsp. of detergent but the average dishwasher only needs 2 tbsp. to clean beautifully. Similarly, the open dispenser is meant to dispense only 1 tbsp. but has an overflow region that makes it easy to put in 2 or even 3 tbsp. Be stingy. Every little bit counts.

"Oops, I Forgot to Use Baking Soda, and the Dishes Are Already in the Dishwasher!"

If you forgot to use the baking soda before loading your dishwasher, go ahead and sprinkle the baking soda on the already-loaded dishes. This method doesn't work as well because the dishes are facing down toward the sprayer and not up where you are sprinkling the soda. Taking a handful of baking soda and tossing it up onto the dishes sort of works. But please, don't use baking soda on your aluminum pots and pans. If left on for very long, the baking soda reacts with the aluminum and discolors it brown or dark gray.

Automatic-Dishwasher Problem Solving

IS YOUR DISHWASHER NOT PERFORMING AS WELL AS IT USED TO, NO MATTER HOW MUCH DETERGENT YOU PUT IN?

When your dishwasher isn't as effective as it used to be, don't waste money by trying to clean your dishes with too much detergent. It's smart to take a little time to take care of a machine that you use every day. I've discovered a few tips that should help yours work and clean better. Follow these easy steps for keeping both you and your dishwasher happy.

1. *Check the bottom of the machine* for accumulated food scraps, bottle caps, labels, broken dishes, or utensils. This kind of stuff can stop the spray arm from getting to all of your dishes. Wait until the machine is off and cooled down, then clean out with a rag or paper towel.
2. *Let your machine run two or three times without any dishes in it.* This will help to clear away any food scraps or other hidden gunk that is stopping it from cleaning.

3. *Dishwashers depend on hot, hot water to clean.* Dishwashers work best when your water heater is set between 140° and 160° Fahrenheit. But many of us have turned our heaters down to 120° or 125° to protect those curious toddlers from accidental burns. If you've turned it down recently or it's cold outside, don't be surprised if the dishes aren't getting as clean. Dishes won't get clean if you run out of hot water, either. Running a load of laundry, turning on the dishwasher, and having two bathrooms' showers on all at once at 6 A.M. may be a little too much for your water heater to take. Dishwashers and laundry machines aren't like those screaming people in the shower telling you that they've run out of hot water. Those machines just go ahead and try to clean no matter what the temperature is.

4. *If after all this your dishwasher still rattles and shakes, give up and call someone to repair it.*

What's the "Best" Way to Load a Dishwasher?

Dishwasher loading was a subject of great dispute among my four sisters and I. Despite the fact that we grew up together, we all seemed to have developed our own unique way of "correctly" loading the dishwasher. Inspired by those often irrational disputes, I've distilled for you the very best of the dishwasher loading tricks.

1. Put those forks and spoons into their little basket with *the handles down*. The spray will reach each individual utensil better, and if their handles are down, the spoons won't nest and stick together. Sort them after they're clean. For safety reasons, *put the pointy knives down*—except for the very thin ones. A thin one can fall through the basket holes and stop the spray arm.

2. Wedge the light items, such as small plastic cups and containers, in the top rack on the far outside edges. Otherwise, they flip over and store water rather than get clean.
3. Put cookie sheets, glass dishes, pie pans, and so on on the bottom rack on the left and right sides. Otherwise, they block the spray from getting to other dishes.
4. Hardened egg stuck on a fork is a notorious dishwashing problem. Tossing all the utensils in a pot or pan filled with water as you clear the table is the time-tested remedy. Give them even a little more time to soak by loading those utensils last.
5. Get an extra dishwasher basket for the top rack of the dishwasher. I got mine for storing baby bottle nipples, but it works great for any small item like caps, small Tupperware tops, measuring spoons, and so forth. If you put these small items in your regular utensil basket, some of them eventually bounce out and fall to the bottom of the machine, reducing your dishwashing power. In older dishwashers, plastic items that fall onto the heating coils can also melt, giving off noxious fumes.
6. Nobody likes to do this, but washing pots and pans by hand makes a lot of sense and in many cases can end up saving time. Get your favorite scrubber, squirt your dishwashing liquid in, and start 'er up. I use baking soda to absorb grease before dipping my sponge into greasy pans, so I don't waste time trying to get the sponge "degreased" before I can do another dish. Pots and pans go straight into the dish rack for open-air drying. This saves the hassle and time of trying to fit those awkward pots and pans into a dishwashing machine that was not designed for them anyway.

◆

Bleaches

What's Really in Them?

Sodium hypochlorite is the scientific name for what we normally refer to as chlorine bleach. Chlorine bleaches, like Clorox, are usually a diluted solution of sodium hypochlorite. Laundry bleaches, such as "all-fabric" bleach or "oxygen" bleaches, usually contain sodium perborate or hydrogen peroxide, washing soda, and detergent. Other bleaches, such as Purex, can contain silicate and washing soda, too.

What Harm Can They Do?

Bleach is the number-one poisonous substance to which children under the age of 6 are exposed.* Bleach is a stomach irritant, and most cases of ingestion just end up with the child simply vomiting, but it can be serious, particularly if it involves a very small child. The fumes can be irritating to the lungs and should generally be avoided by those with respiratory or heart conditions.

"I Use Bleach So Much I Don't Know If I Could Ever Give It Up."

Chlorine bleach is such a handy all-purpose cleaner that you are right to want it around your house. It disinfects, removes stains, makes whites white, even cleans

---

*1993 American Association of Poison Control Centers Report, Washington, D.C.

counters. It's in our drinking water and our swimming pools, so it must be safe, right? Wrong.

Bleach is a very strong chemical and should be used with caution. Too many dangerous accidents happen with bleach for me to have it around the house. Looking at the 1993 and 1994 American Association of Poison Control Centers' annual reports, I was astonished to find out that bleach is involved in the number-one call to Poison Control Centers about children under the age of 6.* And that statistic does not include the exposures related to the mixing of bleach with other chemicals.

But I'm not as against bleach as I sound. For years after I discovered my nontoxic recipes, I kept a small 16-oz. bottle of bleach on the laundry shelf. Just in case, I thought. Whites do get stained and they do need bleaching. Well, I just never used it. I wanted to avoid that irritating bleachy odor you get when you are soaking something. Occasionally, I would be tempted to put a slosh or two in the laundry, but I always felt nervous about ruining my clothes. It's so easy to pour in too much, resulting in holes and white spots. And I've also found out the hard way that bleach damages Spandex. Apparently, the elastic fibers that make that Spandex so nice and stretchy just simply break down in bleach. I ended up giving my bottle of bleach away the next time I moved. I will occasionally use the liquid Clorox 2 bleach, but as I get better at stain control, I find that's not even necessary. Clorox 2 is a nonchlorine oxygen bleach, safe for a variety of fabrics, and easier on the environment than regular chlorine bleach. It also dispenses in a safe, controllable way—not so with your ordinary gallon jug of Clorox.

---

*There were only 250 more personal exposures reported for systemic antibiotics than for bleach.

"But I Use Bleach Regularly in the Wash to Get Out Stains."

Most laundry whites do not need bleaching. It's much more effective to take care of spots and stains as they happen and treat each fabric and stain appropriately. Many people include a chlorine bleach in the wash simply out of habit. Talk to professional cleaners, and they will tell you that the regular use of chlorine bleach in your wash is not suggested. Over time, the chlorine bleach can weaken your fabrics, thus causing unnecessary tears and rips. It's not necessarily good for your washing machine, either. If you use an excessive amount of bleach, it can cause metal parts to corrode and wear out, even causing rust stains on your clothes. Chemical bleaches also give your clothes an unnatural blue tint rather than a true-beauty white. But, dirt, dyes, and permanent stains will fade significantly with bleaching. *Using a chlorine bleach as a spot remover for permanent stains makes sense.* I kept a bottle of bleach around for several years after I switched to nontoxics.

"I'm Not Giving Up My Clorox Yet!"

Remember chlorine bleach is corrosive at a pH of 10.5. Clorox likes to keep their bleaches at pH 10.4 so that you can't technically call them "corrosive." I call that *too tricky* for me. Nevertheless, ordinary bleach can irritate your lungs and skin, and an accidental spill can damage your clothes, your rugs, and your furniture. Imagine if we collected all the clothes that have been ruined by using too much chlorine bleach—what a mountain that would form! Don't forget to add rugs, carpets, and furniture to that mountain, too!

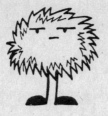

"Okay, I'm Considering Giving It Up. What Can I Use Instead?"

In most situations, you can just do without it. Many people use bleach for stains because they don't know how to handle them. We make simple mistakes, such as letting a stain sit around for hours and hours while it sets, or putting sugar stains in hot water (which actually sets the stain), or trying to remove grass stains with a detergent (detergents can actually make grass stains permanent instead of getting them out). Take a look at the stain-removing tips in my Laundry Detergents section (see pp. 191–205). My tips really work, and you don't need to have a reference manual by your washer to figure it out, either! As I've gotten better at stain removal, I've found that I simply don't need any bleach at all.

If you want to fade a color or a permanent stain, then white vinegar, lemon juice, and sunlight are all mild bleaches you can enjoy using. If want to take out the grays or yellows, then try adding a vinegar rinse at the end of the wash. I keep a couple of gallons of scented white vinegar in my laundry room for this very purpose. I presoak with 1 or more cups. Vinegar, like any bleach, can weaken fabrics so don't use too much. My favorite scent for the laundry is apple. Some dyes and fabrics (like cheap rayons from India) will bleed, so when in doubt, leave it out.

If you do decide to use a commercial bleach, oxygen bleaches are easier on the environment. Choose the all-fabric bleaches that contain sodium perborate or hydrogen peroxide or those labeled as nonchlorine. Clorox 2 is a good example.

What Are the Cleaning Products That Kids Get into Most Often?

In descending order,* here are the cleaning items that children most often get into:

- Bleach
- Laundry detergents
- Disinfectants (mostly the pine-oil ones)
- Furniture polishes
- Wall, floor, and tile cleaners

These are all cleaners that tend to be left on the floor or in other handy places children can reach. That's a good reason to be careful not to leave your cleaners on the floor—and a good reason to use safer, milder cleaners.

Ready for some natural bleach alternatives now?

---

*Approximate order based on 1993 and 1994 American Association of Poison Control Centers Report, Washington, D.C.

Sunny Skies

Bleach Alternative

A Natural Whitener Named After My Favorite Preschool

Ingredients: Sunlight and lemon juice.

What to Do: Everybody knows that blond hair turns brighter in the summer sun. Sunlight is an incredibly powerful and wonderful natural bleach, especially for cotton whites like T-shirts, sheets, blouses, and pants. Old-fashioned as it may sound, leaving your whites and jeans to dry in the sun keeps them fresh and white, or in the case of your jeans, a lovely faded blue. You can use sunlight for spots, too, but try adding a little lemon juice before you set them out in the sun. Be sure to launder after. Sunlight is free, of course, and completely natural. Make use of the beautiful star we live around.

Effectiveness Rating: 60%

Commercial Brand* vs. Sunny Skies (32-oz. laundry bleach): $1.09 vs. free. *Sunlight* is free. If you use the lemon juice as a spot bleach, it will cost you about 2¢ per application. You'll **save** $1.09.

---

*Price comparison with Clorox bleach.

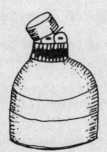

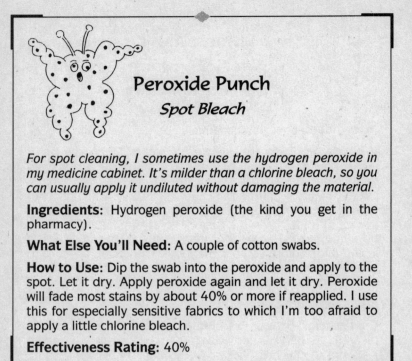

Peroxide Punch
Spot Bleach

For spot cleaning, I sometimes use the hydrogen peroxide in my medicine cabinet. It's milder than a chlorine bleach, so you can usually apply it undiluted without damaging the material.

Ingredients: Hydrogen peroxide (the kind you get in the pharmacy).

What Else You'll Need: A couple of cotton swabs.

How to Use: Dip the swab into the peroxide and apply to the spot. Let it dry. Apply peroxide again and let it dry. Peroxide will fade most stains by about 40% or more if reapplied. I use this for especially sensitive fabrics to which I'm too afraid to apply a little chlorine bleach.

Effectiveness Rating: 40%

Apple Orchard Laundry Rinse
Bleach Alternative

Vinegar is a mild bleach that is safe to use on most fabrics as a laundry rinse, fabric softener, and presoak. I use this recipe to make a presoaking bleach if I have a white that I want brightened. Vinegar can make cheap dyes and fabrics run and fade. If you have any doubt, test it on a small piece of fabric in the sink first.

Ingredients: Apple-scented white distilled vinegar.

How to Make: To scent the vinegar, add about 25 drops of apple fragrance to a gallon jug of vinegar.

How to Use: Put your laundry in the machine during the pre-soak cycle. Add 1 or more cups of vinegar and let the laundry soak. Vinegar brightens your whites and bleaches only very mildly. It *deodorizes* with a punch.

Effectiveness Rating as a Bleach: 40%

Effectiveness Rating as a Deodorizer: 100%

Car Cleaners

What's Really in Them?

Car cleaning involves the full range of different chemical cleaners: detergents for the exterior, petroleum distillate-based vinyl protectors, water-polluting engine cleaners, and extremely hazardous acid-based chrome and mag wheel cleaners.

I've simplified car cleaning to just the basic nontoxics.

How to Wash Your Car Nontoxically

A BUCKET OF SUDS

A bucket of water and 2 tbsp. of a hand-dishwashing liquid detergent are all you really need to make the outside of your car shiny and clean. I use Dr. Bronner's Sal Suds. Detergents work great for degreasing and getting rid of tough road dirt. Only 2 tbsp. of the hand-dishwashing detergent and 3 tbsp. of the Sal Suds, please. It's easy to want to use more, but you don't really need it.

SODA CHROME

Use a baking-soda paste and a white nylon-backed sponge on the chrome. If you've got oodles of bugs, sprinkle soda, spray with water, and let sit for a few minutes or more to loosen those doodles. Rub and rinse with water. For a nice shine, be sure to rinse again. It's best to use Club Clean™ for the final rinse. Buff shiny with a soft cloth. To remove rust, put on a paste of salt and lemon juice and let sit. Rub with the rind of the lemon. Rust is gone.

GIVE YOUR LEATHER SEATS THE NATURAL OLIVE OIL TREATMENT

You can use the It's A Lotsa Polish™ recipe of olive oil and vinegar for your leather interior. Use a little less vinegar than you would for the regular formula. Apply sparingly and rub in thoroughly to avoid oil stains on your clothes.

SPARKLING WINDOWS

Use Club Clean™ for the windows and inside glass. Have you ever noticed that after your car has been in the sun for a while, the inside windows have a thin, sticky, transparent film on them? That film is the chemical outgassing from the vinyls, glues, and upholstery in your car interior. I don't know why this is the case, but my tests showed that Club Clean™ was more effective at removing those chemical residues than any commercial glass cleaner I tested. Simpler is better.

A SUPER TIRE SCRUB

Scrub tires with a brush and the Earth Scrub™ recipe (see p. 239) made with liquid hand-dishwashing detergent. While you are at it, use the scrub to clean your headlights, too. Let the scrub soak surfaces with baked-on bugs, rinse well with water, and finish-rinse with Club Clean™.

CLEANING THE BATTERY TERMINALS

Cleaning off those rusting battery terminals not only will make them look nice but will also make them last longer. Make a paste of three parts baking soda to one part water: 1½ cups of soda with ½ cup of water is a good amount. Unhook the cables, scrub with the paste, wipe clean, and rehook the cables. Apply petroleum jelly to prevent future rusting, and you're done.

Buff and Shine

Nontoxic Substitute for Products Such as Armor-All

Petroleum jelly is a simple, safer substance to protect your car seats and dashboard. Petroleum jelly will condition and nourish the vinyl and other assorted plastic parts. Put a small glob on your rag and buff it in. Don't use too much. I repeat: don't use too much, or you will attract dirt and dust. It works great on tires, too. But be careful not to get *any* on glass or windows. It smears and streaks terribly!

Commercial Brand* vs. Petroleum Jelly (16-oz. vinyl protector and cleaner): $7.36 vs. $2.09. A jar of petroleum jelly should cost you about $2. You'll **save** $5.27.

---

*Price comparison with Armor-All.

Crazy Mom's* Car Cleaning Kit™
Car Cleaners in a Kit

This car kit makes me invincible on the road. When we bought a new car, I kept having visions of my daughter throwing up in it. She had thrown up in our other car just 2 weeks earlier. How was I going to keep this car nice and still let my daughter in it? Necessity is the mother of invention, so I created the Crazy Mom's Car Cleaning Kit™. Now, I'm ready. So many times, I have needed just a little squirt and a wipe to clean that little baby face and those little hands right up. Somehow, it's always at the last minute in the car before we get to Grandma's and Grandpa's house that I notice how dirty Sophie's gotten.

Ingredients: Club soda, liquid soap, and scented vinegar.

What Else You'll Need: A small tool box–size plastic bin (art-supply bins work great) with a handle, two 8-oz. spray-bottles, an 8-oz. squirt-bottle, and four small, good cleaning rags (washcloth size).

How to Make: I bought an art-bin box at an office-supply store for $7.99. It has a handle on it and fits right under the seat. Inside it, I put a small spray-bottle of club soda–glass cleaner, a small squirt-bottle of apple-scented vinegar and water, and a small spray-bottle of diluted peppermint-scented liquid soap along with four cotton terry cloth rags. If you have room in the box and you have leather seats, you might want to include a small bottle of Lotsa Leather, too (see pp. 152).

How to Use: Use liberally for daily car-cleaning emergencies. Remember to turn the spray-bottles to the off position as you put them back into the car kit. It's helpful to have the cleaner in the bottle rather than in the car kit itself. And don't forget to bring this kit inside the house for regular cleaner refills and new, clean rags. It's a drag to need the kit and not have any cleaner left.

Effectiveness Rating: 100%

*To give the proper credit to the daddies, grandmas, grandpas, stepdads and step-moms, baby-sitters, teachers, and nannies of the world: the *Mom* in Crazy Mom's Car Kit™ refers to anyone who takes care of a child, be they male or female, old or young.

Here are some of the many ways my family has used Crazy Mom's Car Cleaning Kit™:

- The first time I used it was when my daughter dumped her bottle on the seat and the milk leaked out onto the beautiful new upholstered seat. I had always feared that old sour-milk car smell. Not this time. As soon as I stopped the car, I grabbed the apple-scented vinegar out of my handy kit and washed it right out. The seat smelled great right away, and the vinegar was convenient and quick. There was no annoying residue milk odor or stain.

- We were on our way home from Yosemite National Park. The car had been sitting in the parking lot for 3 days without use and was very dusty. When we got in the car, we could hardly see out the front windows. Nobody wanted to make an extra trip to the gas station to clean the windows. We just wanted to get home. I suggested that we clean them up with the club soda in the car kit. The rags were filthy when my husband finished with the windows, but he had a smile on his face. Now we could go home.

- Burger King stop for a children's meal and a toy: my daughter, Sophie, wants to hold the soda all by herself. I'm tired and I relent. Of course, the inevitable happens—sugary soda everywhere. Stop. Sophie's clothes come off. I squirt-clean her hands and body with the soap and water, then rinse the floor with some club soda. More soap and water. Final vinegar rinse. Spray-clean assorted sugary drips on the interior. Relax. Thank you, Crazy Mom's.

- It was a very long (5-hour) car trip with my toddler—5 hours is a *very* long time when you are only 2. Near the end of the ride, it was hot and we were all cranky and tired. Sophie looked like our car, dusty and dirty. I whipped out the club soda cleaner and started spraying. She loved it. We took her socks off and sprayed her feet with the club soda. She giggled. Then she got hold of the club soda and Mommy got wet. This small spray-bottle of soda entertained and refreshed us for the last crucial hour home.

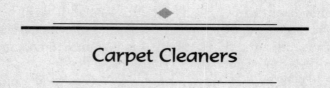

Carpet Cleaners

What's Really in Them?

Ingredients in carpet cleaners include ethanol, ammonia, detergents, and fragrances. Carpet spot removers can contain perchloroethylene, naphthalene, and trichloroethylene.

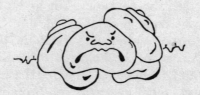

What Harm Can They Do?

The strong fragrances used in carpet cleaners can irritate those with sensitivities. Spot cleaners are among the most dangerous and can irritate the skin and are often poisonous when ingested.

Keeping your carpet clean is probably more important than you realize. Dust and dirt grind and wear away carpets faster than you think. The dirt isn't good to breathe, either. Studies have shown that in more than 75% of the homes tested, rug dust contains high mutagenic and/or toxic levels of chemicals.* Toddlers ingest 2.5 times as much carpet dust as adults since they sit and play on carpets, and because they are smaller, their risk is even greater.

Steam-cleaning is really the best thing you can do for your carpet. The hot, hot water kills fleas, dust mites, and any other bacteria that may be causing odors. But it's expensive, and, even though we'd like to, we can't do it every month, so here's how to handle those spills, spots, and odors in the meantime.

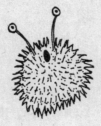

*Roberts, John W., M.Sc., and Gulyn Warren, Ph.D. "Sources of Toxics in House Dust." *International Journal of Biosocial Research* 9 (1987), 82–91.

Cornmeal Carpet Mop
Carpet Spill Absorber

What's a carpet without a spill? A magic one! In real life, we live with spills. Here's what to do when you get a nasty one.

Ingredients: Cornmeal.

What Else You'll Need: A vacuum or carpet sweeper.

How to Use: To sop up big liquid spills quickly, you can use cornmeal. I keep a box handy in the kitchen. Dump cornmeal directly onto the spill. Allow 5–15 minutes for the meal to sop up the spill. Sweep the mess into a dustpan and discard. Vacuum up the remaining meal. Then I use a little squirt of Go Spot Go™ (see recipe on pp. 200–01) to get the remaining stain. Rinse with vinegar and sop up with old towels. Emergency's over!

Effectiveness Rating: 60%

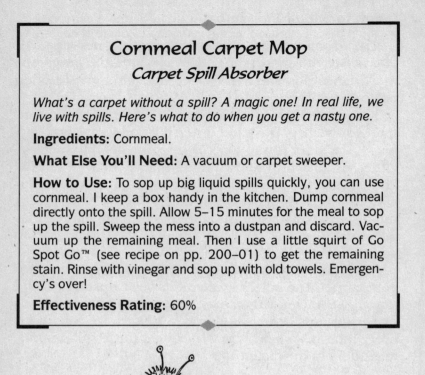

Soda Lightful
Carpet Deodorizer

Scented baking soda is an excellent carpet deodorizer, but you'll pay a premium for it in the grocery store. It's easy to make it for yourself at home for pennies.

Ingredients: A scented baking soda.

What Else You'll Need: A vacuum or carpet sweeper.

How to Use: Sprinkle the baking soda on any area of your carpet that needs deodorizing. Let sit for a couple of hours—overnight if it really needs deodorizing. Vacuum. I don't like any powder residue, so I like to finish up with a peppermint-scented vinegar rinse. I squirt on the vinegar and then put some old towels down and stomp on them to soak it up. Your carpet will smell fresh and clean! This is also an easy way to freshen up a small area rug or carpet.

Effectiveness Rating: 75%–80%

Foam Alone
Carpet Cleaner

What do I do for general carpet cleaning? Here's an easy way to clean up the ever-present spots of food, juice, and soda.

Ingredients: Liquid soap or detergent.

What Else You'll Need: A blender.

How to Use: Put $1/4$ cup liquid soap or detergent in a blender with $1/3$ cup water or more. Blend until foamy. Smear the mixture on the carpet spots and let it sit for a few minutes—or longer if dirtier. If you have a good carpet brush, use it. They really work. I finish with a squirt of vinegar and sop up the excess with some old towels.

Effectiveness Rating: 70%

What's quiet as a mouse, saves on your electricity bill, fits in the smallest of closets, is easy to carry up and down stairs, has no cords to tangle or fray, is safe enough for children to use, never needs any bags, won't wake up or scare the baby, doesn't blow dust into the air, is inexpensive, and lasts for 20 years or more?

Answer: a good old-fashioned carpet sweeper.

Why don't more department stores carry carpet sweepers? I don't know, but they are missing out by not offering a great product. Get one. See the catalog companies in my Resources section (see pp. 283–89). They also make thoughtful baby-shower gifts. How many new parents have awakened their baby with that noisy old vacuum? I use my carpet sweeper all the time to pick up those endless, everyday baby spills, such as peas, crackers, Cheerios, and Play-Doh pieces. When I was in high school, I used to sell a pretty red carpet sweeper when I went door to door selling Fuller brush products to earn money for college. Maybe that's why I feel so comfortable selling cleaning products to you—early training.

◆

Disinfectants

What's Really in Them?

Disinfectants can contain quaternary ammonium compounds such as the popular benzalkonium chloride, pine oil, alcohol, ethanol, phenol or derivatives of phenol (*o*-phenyl phenol), cresol, TCE, PDCBs, butyl cellosolve, detergents, and formaldehyde.

What Harm Do They Do?

Disinfectant ingredients are designed to kill germs, so they're often toxic in nature because of this "killing" aspect. A disinfectant may not *seem* harmful to humans if diluted or exposure is limited. But, historically speaking, there have been several incidents where a chemical disinfectant had been thought to be okay for use and then its toxicity was discovered.

Disinfectants are known to be quite irritating to the eyes, skin, and particularly the nose. Concentrated solutions of quaternary ammonium compounds can destroy the mucous membranes. It's surprising how much chemical we can absorb by simply breathing the fumes in an enclosed area.

Disinfectants can also destroy the balance in your septic system and make it difficult for the treatment of your water waste. In a landfill, they can inhibit any natural composting action, and the runoff of the chemicals can pollute streams and poison fish and other aquatic life. Many disinfectants contain ingredients that are federally classified as hazardous and should not be thrown into the ordinary trash. They should be used up or poured down the drain with lots of water.

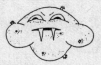

All quaternary ammonium compounds can be toxic. Ingestion can cause burns in the throat. Phenols and cresols are especially toxic. Although many companies have phased out these chemicals in disinfectants, you can still find them in some older formulations. All phenols are corrosive and damaging to the skin and eyes, and prolonged exposure can lead to liver and kidney damage.

THE CASE OF DISINFECTANT SPRAYS

Disinfectant sprays like Lysol are particularly deceiving because many people try to use them to disinfect and freshen the air. If you look closely at the can, Lysol is recommended for use *on surfaces only*. Any disinfectant is effective at killing those germs for only a very short time. A few minutes later, more germs will come flying out of a coughing mouth or sneezing nose. Most health experts agree that one of the best ways to control air-borne viruses is to open a window! Consumer Reports Books says: "It's really not possible to prevent the spread of germs in the house by using a disinfectant." In addition, the active ingredients in many spray disinfectants are registered pesticides, and the ethanol (alcohol) they are suspended in is known to be irritating to the eyes, nose, and throat. Do we really need to spray little bits of pesticide and alcohol in the air just to make sure we don't spread germs to each other? To reduce the spreading of germs, most doctors recommend (especially for children) *fresh air; frequent hand washing; the washing of toys, telephones, or other frequently touched items; and the isolation of the sick from the healthy.*

Isn't It Important to Disinfect When We Clean?

Maybe we don't really need to super-disinfect. Antiseptics were life-saving developments for wartime wounds and peacetime surgeries. Keeping germs under control in medical and hospital settings can make a significant difference between life and death. But most germs can't be controlled because the majority of them are airborne, constantly reproducing or renewed, and always invisibly transferred. That's why hospitals are hothouses of disease. Hospital-related diseases and deaths are common, particularly in the elderly. Modern science hasn't gotten rid of germs, disease, or death. No wonder we're still scared of germs.

But we live with germs; we breathe germs and eat germs. Some are bad, but some are also very, very good. If we killed off all the germs we live with, we would get very, very sick. Staying healthy may have a lot more to do with living a balanced, natural life (pure foods, clean air, water, and rest) than with killing off "dangerous" germs.

Cleaning companies use the word *disinfectant* on their product labels because it seems to have such a magical power to get you to *buy*. The practical reality of disinfecting is this: in most cases, hot or warm water, a cleaner (a soap, detergent, and/or mild abrasive), and some good "mechanical action" is all you really need! *It's the frequency and regularity of cleaning that probably has the most significant health effect.*

But what about toilets? What about those icky, moldy, bacteria-filled places? What about food surfaces, sick rooms, garbage, toilet overflows, urine, animal and human feces? It's important to have a disinfecting cleaner for these tasks, something that gets things superclean and has extra germ-killing action. I like to use the natural tea tree oil as an alternative disinfecting agent in my cleaners. Derived from the tea tree found in the outbacks of Australia, this oil has the remarkable qualities of being a powerful antiseptic without the usually associated toxicity. Known as the first-aid kit in a bottle, it is an excellent antiseptic. It smells superclean and works great with all my recipes. I've found it's all I really need.

IS TEA TREE OIL REALLY A DISINFECTANT?

Tea tree oil is *in the process* of being registered as a disinfectant in this country. So we can't quite legally say it is a disinfectant yet! But it has been known for many years in Australia as an excellent disinfectant. No matter what the claims are, you can still get the same wonderful tea tree oil at your local health-food store. If you take the Australian's word for it, you, too, can enjoy its antigerm qualities.

Following are my solutions to the disinfecting problems in the house. **Note:** I call the following recipes "disinfectant alternatives" because the government has strict regulations about what you can and cannot call a "disinfectant" commercially. These recipes are alternatives to the commercial disinfectants that you might find in the store, and, although not necessarily "disinfectants" themselves, they may be disinfectant-like in their properties. But as with any disinfectant, be sure to label it properly: list all the ingredients and include a warning to keep out of the reach of children.

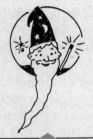

Merlin's Magic™
Antiseptic Soap Spray

This recipe takes advantage of the magical antiseptic power of tea tree oil.

Ingredients: Liquid soap, purified water, and tea tree oil.

What Else You'll Need: A 16-oz. squirt- or spray-bottle.

How to Make: Fill the bottle almost full with water and *then* add 3 tbsp. of liquid soap to prevent the bottle from sudsing up as you fill. Because minerals inhibit the cleaning action of soap, it's best to use purified or distilled water for this recipe, especially if you have hard water. Add 20–30 drops or more of tea tree oil for antiseptic power. Shake to mix. I like to use unscented or eucalyptus-scented liquid soap for this recipe.

How to Use: Squirt this wonderfully safe alternative on floors, laundry, toys, doorknobs, bathtubs, toilet seats, and more. I've used it to clean up after the nasties like urine, toilet bowl overflows, vomit, and more unmentionables. Some of you will love the superclean medicinal smell of tea tree oil; some of you won't. Use Merlin's Magic™ to wash those little hands, too. It's a refreshing alternative to those expensive antibacterial soaps.

Effectiveness Rating: 95%

Commercial Brand* vs. Merlin's Magic™ (28-oz. antiseptic soap spray): $2.99 vs. $1.10. 5 tbsp. of Dr. Bronner's soap is 60¢, and you'll use 50¢ worth of tea tree oil. You'll **save** $1.89 each time you refill the bottle.

---

*Price comparison with Lysol spray.

Crocodile Clean™
Disinfectant Alternative

Tea tree oil–ed vinegar?! I've used this for tasks such as cleaning the laundry-room floor of mice smells, rinsing out picnic garbage cans, and treating smelly outside concrete. Vinegar is also known to have some germ-killing power, too!

Ingredients: White distilled vinegar and tea tree oil.

What Else You'll Need: You can use the solution straight from the gallon jug of vinegar or put it in a 16-oz. squirt-bottle.

How to Make: To make the scented vinegar, add ½ tsp. or more (1 dropperful or 50 drops) of tea tree oil to a gallon of vinegar. When measuring the tea tree oil, don't use plastic measuring spoons! The oil will dissolve them. Use metal teaspoons or estimate ¼ of a teaspoon by using a regular dinner spoon. Droppers are the best. Fill the squirt-bottle with the tea tree oil vinegar if you like, or just use it directly from the jug.

How to Use: Use this disinfectant alternative rinse anywhere, on floors, walls, pails, tubs. I'm sloppy about using this recipe and just usually slosh a bunch of tea tree oil–scented vinegar wherever I want to clean. I let it sit for a few minutes, scrub, and squirt with a little soap and water if needed, slosh on some more vinegar, maybe rinse with water, and the smelly job is done!

Effectiveness Rating: 75%

Commercial Brand* vs. Crocodile Clean™ (17-oz. disinfectant alternative): $2.79 vs. 67¢. 17 oz. of vinegar costs about 17¢; add 50¢ worth of tea tree oil. You'll **save** $2.12.

---

*Price comparison with Lysol disinfectant (liquid).

Doctor Diaper Pail
Disinfecting Spray Alternative

Some people like to spray disinfectants in their diaper pails to control odors. I developed this recipe to help keep those diaper odors down, but it makes a great cleaner, too!

Ingredients: Baking soda and tea tree oil; perhaps some lemon and lavender oil, too.

What Else You'll Need: A shaker container.

How to Make: Add ½ tsp. (one dropperful or 50 drops) of tea tree oil to 1 cup of baking soda. Stir and work out lumps with a fork. Don't use plastic measuring spoons to measure the oil, or the oil will dissolve them. Metal teaspoons work fine. Estimating the amount of oil roughly and pouring it directly from the bottle into the shaker is neater. Using a dropper is best.

How to Use: Sprinkle some of this antiseptic baking soda in the bottom of the diaper pail or on top of the diapers to help absorb those odors. You can also use this power powder to clean out the pail. For a sweeter smell, scent your baking soda with a mixture of lemon, lavender, and tea tree oil. Both lemon and lavender are supposed to have antiseptic powers as well. I've used the mixture for the tub and toilet, too. It's terrific.

Effectiveness Rating: 60%

What Really Needs Disinfecting in My House?

There are few areas in the house that need disinfecting: the cutting board, the toilet, the garbage can, kitchen sponges, and those ubiquitous little germy hands. Most of these can be adequately cleaned with hot water and soap.

THE CUTTING BOARD

The cutting board is one of the few areas in our homes that truly needs disinfecting (see my suggestions for this in the Kitchen Cleansers section, pp. 184–91). Cutting boards could be a source of food poisoning more often than you think. Bugs can grow quickly in meats, turkey, and fish. What you thought was the 24-hour flu could have been from the leftover turkey that was left out too long. Rubbing a little bit of salt and water into your board and rinsing it off does an excellent job of disinfecting your board after cutting meats.* Lemon juice and salt, or a little vinegar, helps to clean and deodorize, too.

THE TOILET

Nobody likes to clean the toilet. Cleaning a toilet is essentially a humbling event. If you are having ego clashes at work, get down and clean a toilet. It will do your soul good. Most of us try to get someone else to do it or just don't do it at all. I counteract my aversion to cleaning toilets by scenting my toilet bowl cleaner with peppermint or tea tree oil. Adding a fresh scent to your cleaner can inspire you to complete the task. I use a spray-bottle of Merlin's Magic™ (see p. 114) tea tree oil–scented soap and water to clean the seats, cover, outside,

---

*This method has not been scientifically proven to disinfect.

and base. Then I flush the toilet, turn off the water just as it drains out, and squirt in one of my tub and tile cleaners. Swish with the toilet brush, turn the water back on, squirt on some scented vinegar to rinse and deodorize, and that's all. *Believe it or not, often it's not the bowl of the toilet that can be the dirtiest. Watch out for the nasties on the base, under the rim, and underneath the seat.* Clean those areas last and toss that rag or sponge right into a bucket for laundering. Please, don't use that rag to clean the rest of the bathroom.

THE GARBAGE CAN

Discarded food is a great place for odors and bacteria to grow. Keep the garbage can lined and emptied out before it starts to smell. To keep your can smelling fresh and clean, throw a handful of scented baking soda in at the bottom. You can also avoid a lot of garbage smells by composting your food waste. I have a separate can for my food waste. It's a small white one that I can open with a foot lever. That's where we dump leftover food and vegetable waste. The inner can lifts right out and gets dumped into the compost every other morning and then rinsed and dried before it goes back. You may not be ready to compost yet, but your city government would be happy if you did! Food waste in the garbage prevents a lot of good stuff from being reclaimed and recycled. Most cities don't reclaim a lot of stuff yet, but watch for it in the future. Cities are running out of landfill space rapidly and are actively looking for solutions.

KITCHEN SPONGES

Kitchen sponges and rags can harbor an extraordinary amount of germs. My rule of thumb is that if it smells, it probably needs disinfecting. The trick is getting the courage to put your nose up to it! Babies and toddlers would tell you—if they could—how disgustingly smelly those kitchen rags are. Even day-old kitchen rags can stink, depending on what they've been up to wiping. What about the ones that haven't been washed in a week? The easiest way to "disinfect" a kitchen rag or sponge is to throw it into the dishwasher. The hot, hot water of the dishwasher will thoroughly disinfect it. I have found that ever since I've been using my baking-soda cleanser at the kitchen sink, my sponges just don't get so smelly anymore. Perhaps the baking soda is keeping those microorganisms away.

LITTLE HANDS EVERYWHERE

A toddler in the house brings home every germ imaginable. I am especially careful about the spread of germs in the winter. Otherwise, we get sick, and then we get sick again and again. *Fresh air and frequent hand washing helps a lot.* If someone is sick in the house, I spray-clean with Merlin's Magic™ (see p. 114) anyplace that we frequently touch: the phone, refrigerator, doorknobs, drawer handles, light switches, and chair arms. Kissing is another great way to spread those germs, but we just can't seem to control it. It's pretty futile when my husband comes home and we all get into a kissing fest. Oh well, so much for germ control.

"I've Heard a Lot About Using a 10-to-1 Solution of Bleach to Disinfect. Should This Be Used At Home?"

Hospitals use a solution of 10 parts water to 1 part bleach to disinfect. It kills the AIDS virus and other serious disease-causing germs. Personally, I don't think it's necessary to superdisinfect like this in the home. Good cleaning habits probably have the most significant effect on maintaining the health of your family.

PREVENTIVE MEASURES

Here's the list of things that I think that actually make a difference in your family's health.

- Keep moist areas clean and dry. Molds and mildews can trigger allergic reactions that you might mistake for a cold.
- Disinfect your cutting board after cutting meats (by rinsing, soaping, and/or salting). And keep foods (especially turkey, fish, and mayonnaise) refrigerated. Kitchen bacteria is a source of food poisoning more often than you might think.
- Wash your hands (especially after changing diapers), and wash your kids' hands. Germs go from hand to mouth in minutes, even in adults.
- Empty the garbage often. This discourages pests and odors. Composting your food waste right away is even better!
- Open the windows. Indoor air pollutants may be having a more significant effect on your health than you think. Opening the windows clears out airborne bacteria and viruses, too!
- Keep your house as humid as possible in the winter. Dry air irritates the respiratory system, making you more susceptible to colds and disease. In the winter, I boil a pot of water with some cinnamon sticks and cloves in it. One pot of water can humidify your house quicker than you might think.

◆

Drain Cleaners

What's Really in Them?

Ingredients in drain cleaners include lye (sodium hydroxide), bleach (sodium hypochlorite), sulfuric acid, hydrochloric acid, and ammonia. Drain cleaners are particularly hazardous because they contain *concentrated* forms of lye, bleach, or ammonia. They can also contain TCE, the ubiquitous air and water pollutant and common dry-cleaning solvent.

What Harm Can They Do?

Drain-cleaning crystals are the worst. Red Devil drain opener (crystals) contains over 95% lye (sodium hydroxide) and has a pH of 14. Crystal Drano is 54% lye (sodium hydroxide). Liquid-Plumr is only about 2% lye but includes 5%–10% sodium hypochlorite (the diluted chemical in laundry bleach). Swallowing a drain cleaner can cause death or dissolve important parts of your body like your mouth, face, and throat. To add insult to injury, they often don't even unclog drains! Everybody knows how dangerous drain cleaners are. They are even used to commit suicide. Ugh.

Why are we hooked on the chemical way? Professional plumbers hate them because they make their job more difficult and dangerous. Explosions can occur as the clog is dissolving, causing the drain cleaner to splash back onto unsuspecting humans! I've talked to plumbers who have scars on their arms from such explosions. Another dangerous scenario is that people put chemical drain cleaner down the drain; it doesn't work, so they start pumping the drain with a plunger, not realizing they are dealing with an extremely hazardous chemical. The drain cleaner accidentally splashes into their eyes, and they end up in the hospital. Their vision is sometimes permanently clouded.

No one I know of recommends the use of those hazardous chemical drain cleaners—no book, no plumber, no cleaning professional. In fact, they all advise against the use of these chemical decloggers! The manual methods of plungers, snakes, motorized drain openers, pressurized air guns, and garden-hose bladders are far more effective, relatively inexpensive, and safe.

Consumer Reports Books has this to say about drain cleaners: "To say that you should use these products with extreme caution is an *understatement*. It's best not to use chemical drain openers at all."

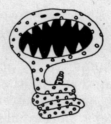

THE TRUTH ABOUT LYE

One afternoon, I was over at the local ecology information center bragging about my safe and amazing alternative recipes. One of the shopkeepers nearby smiled and said, "I think that's a great idea," and proceeded to tell me her tragic story. When she was a small child, she accidentally swallowed drain cleaner. Drain cleaner is truly one of the worst things for your child to get into. It contains sodium hydroxide, commonly known as lye, which will dissolve skin and tissue on contact. Even a few crystals on wet skin can cause damage. When a child actually swallows it, it is serious business. In this woman's case, she lost most of the tissue in her mouth, and her cheeks and face were severely disfigured. As a child, she was teased incessantly because of her looks. Only later on as a teenager could she have the cosmetic surgery needed. Her face is still quite scarred today.

Why Are Chemical Drain Cleaners Still on the Shelves?

Chemical drain cleaners are not only dangerous to you and potentially damaging to your plumbing, but often they don't even work. Consumer Reports Books rates most chemical drain cleaners at the bottom of their list. Many people pour cleaners into their drains only to have them sit as dangerous, toxic pools in their tub or sink until the plumber arrives.

Why are these products still on the market? It is extremely difficult to legally remove any product from the store shelves. Drain cleaners stay there mostly because we keep buying them. Why? Because of the power of their advertising, their image. It's actually the idea that they will work that sells them, not the reality.

Important: Do not use any nontoxic unclogging methods *after* having used a chemical drain cleaner. You poured the chemical down, and now it must be handled with caution. Call a professional.

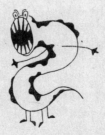

"My Drain Is Really Clogged and I Don't Want to Have to Call a Plumber. What Can I Do?"

If your sink is clogged, first evaluate the situation. Most clogs are from hair, oils, dried-up soap, and other gunk. The best way to unclog this type is *manually*, not chemically. You just want to push or pull and get that gunk out. If more than one sink or tub is backed up, then you have a deep clog, and you should probably call a plumber—now. Otherwise, try these easy tips.

Here are seven steps to unclog the drain the safe way:

1. If there is a sink trap (a small metal strainer) in the drain, pull it out and clean it. Use scissors to cut the tightly wrapped hairs and then pull them out. If you like, clean the strainer with a little bit of baking soda and then soak for 5 to 10 minutes in vinegar to help dissolve the gunk. Rinse well and replace.

2. Use a plunger. If necessary, plug the overflow opening with a wet rag. Fill the area up with enough water to cover the top of the plunger. Make sure the seal on the plunger is tight. Using some petroleum jelly on the rim will help, especially if it is a toilet clog. You can also get special plungers to fit the toilet. Push, pull, push, pull—at least 10 times, lifting the plunger up quickly on the last pull. Repeat several times before giving up. If this sounds like too athletic of a job for you, then enlist someone with a strong set of arms.

3. If you suspect a simple hair, soap, oil clog, bend a metal coat hanger with pliers into a probing loop. Use the loop to try to pull out enough hair and other gunk from the drain to get the water flowing so that you can rinse down the rest of the clog. If you suspect metal objects down the drain (like hair clips, rings, utensils, etc.) get a magnet that will fit down the drain, tie some heavy-duty string or wire around it, and go fishing!

4. If you've got a greasy garbage disposal clog, try my Lemon Iced recipe (see p. 74). If your disposal is jammed, then turn off the disposal, put in a wooden stick or handle (broomstick or spoon), and pushing it against one of the metal ledges at the bottom of the disposal, rotate it counterclockwise. Remove the stick. Turn on the disposal again to see if it has been unclogged.

5. Try a plumber's snake. They are inexpensive and easy to use; you can find one at your local hardware store. The kind that wind up into a canister are good. You could also pick up a bacterial drain opener if you want to try one out. The snake is a smarter purchase. It is more effective and will be there waiting for you the next time you have a clog. Remove the trap or strainer. Thread the snake in slowly, rotating it continuously. When you feel the clog, pull the snake out carefully. Clean and rinse. If the drain is still clogged, repeat again.

6. Pour ½ cup baking soda, ½ cup salt, and ½ cup water down the drain. Let the mixture sit overnight. Rinse well with boiling water. Try the plunger again. Too much salt for too long can do damage to your pipes, so use this recipe with discretion.

7. Okay, you've got a serious clog. If you are like me, you will call a plumber now. If you are the determined handy-dandy type, continue reading. Go to the hardware store again and ask the person at the counter what he or she has for clearing a drain. The clerk will be able to help you the best for your particular situation. You can rent large, motorized snakes if your drain really needs it or try a pressure-air gun or garden-hose bladder. You can also try taking off the trap under the sink or toilet. Be sure to put an empty bucket underneath before removing the trap so as to catch the water that will come gushing out. Don't do

as the last guy who came in to fix our clogged garbage disposal did. He forgot the bucket, and all that gooky water soaked and dirtied my cleaning products under the sink. Never, ever open the trap if you have already poured in corrosive commercial drain cleaner.

When all else fails, call a plumber and promise yourself to prevent the clog next time.

Drain Clogs: An Ounce of Prevention Is Worth a Pound of Cure

- *In the kitchen*, never pour grease down a drain or garbage disposal. Pour warm (not hot!) grease into a paper cup and put in the garbage instead. And, use lots of *hot* water to rinse greasy foods down the disposal. Don't put piles of potato peels or shifty rice down that disposal, either!
- *In the shower and tub*, use a drain trap to catch hair and clean it out regularly.
- *In the bathroom*, don't flush disposable diapers, sanitary napkins, or tampons down the toilet. Wrap these items up in toilet paper and put them in the trash instead. You can also use toilet lid locks to keep the toys out and keep your toddler safe. The Right Start mail-order company offers an easy-to-install one (no tools or screws needed) for $9.95. The company's phone number is (800) 548-8531.
- *In the garage or basement*, don't sweep dirt and other clogging items down the drain thinking they will just disappear—they won't.
- *Install strainers on your drains*. My sister has the wonderful old-fashioned type that are circular and just sit over the drain. They're easy to pick up and clean.

Toys in the Toilet?

Why do kids like to throw toys in the toilet? I certainly don't know why but they do. What do you do when they've clogged the toilet? Fish them out, of course. There are specially designed toilet snakes just to help you out. Mr. Bob, a loving and friendly preschool administrator for 27 years, turned me on to the Toilet Cleaner by Cobra, which is available at the hardware store for only $7.99. Now, that's a whole lot better than the price of a plumber! Follow the instructions on the package, and those toys will get pushed down the pipe or just come popping out. This works about 50% of the time.

Fizz 'N' Free™

Drain Cleaner

This is an easy and entertaining way to keep your drains clear, clean, and odor-free. It's only somewhat effective at clearing a clog, but it is a truly great way to prevent them.

Ingredients: Baking soda and scented vinegar.

How to Make: Use the baking soda and white distilled vinegar right from their store-bought containers. There's nothing to make, except for perhaps a scented vinegar (see scented vinegar recipes, pp. 252–55).

What to Do: Pour about ½ cup of baking soda into the drain. Add a cup or more of white vinegar. The mixture will start to fizz. Cover the drain with a stopper or plunger for a couple of minutes until the fizzing stops. The bubbles work to clean the drain. Rinse well with hot or boiling water. Repeat again if necessary.

How to Use: This helps to *prevent* clogged drains and may work on only very mild clogs. For serious clogs, see my seven ways to unclog your drains (see pp. 124–26). *Never* ever use this recipe after you have used a commercial drain cleaner!

You have an extremely dangerous chemical in your drain, and you need to call a plumber to handle it properly.

Effectiveness Rating: 40%

Commercial Brand* vs. Fizz 'N' Free™ (16-oz. drain cleaner): $2.79 vs. 39¢. ½ cup of baking soda costs 15¢; 1½ cups of vinegar costs 24¢. You'll **save** $2.40 each time you refill the bottle.

---

*Price comparison with Drāno.

La Bomba
Drain Unclogger

In my book, many of the old-fashioned ways are still the best.

What You'll Need: A plunger, petroleum jelly, and a wet rag.

How to Use: I suppose some people don't use plungers because you have to push and pull and chemicals seem easier. Despite the effort you have to put into using plungers, they really work. Plug up that overflow opening with a wet rag first and fill the sink or tub up with enough water to cover the top of the plunger. You also need a good seal. Cover the rim of the plunger with a thick layer of petroleum jelly, squish, push, and pull, and the clog is gone!

Effectiveness Rating: 75%

Commercial Brand* vs. La Bomba (32-oz. drain cleaner): $3.89 vs. $1.10, which is the amortized cost of the plunger at 55¢ per use (if you use it only 10 times in its life span, compared with two uses in one bottle of drain opener. You'll **save** $2.79.

---

*Price comparison with Liquid-Plumr.

Fabric Softeners

What's Really in Them?

Ingredients in fabric softeners can include alkyl diethyl ammonium chloride, synthetic fragrances, and detergents.

What Harm Can They Do?

Commercial fabric softeners can't do much harm, although they could be dangerous if ingested in a large amount; but they almost never are. A more significant factor is what I consider the air-polluting effect of those smelly fabric softener sheets. You can hardly walk down the street without sniffing those dryer perfumes. For those of us who are sensitive to chemicals, it can be quite annoying.

Some Fabric Softener Facts

1. Dryer sheets, such as Bounce, Snuggle, and Cling Free, often use inexpensive scents to mask the chemical smells of their ingredients (no wonder I've always disliked them). If you wouldn't use a cheap perfume, why should your laundry?
2. You may think you need fabric softening when actually, you are just sensitive to the detergent residues in your clothes. Detergent residues can make your clothes feel rough and your skin itchy and dry. Instead, get rid of those residues by using less detergent or adding vinegar to your rinse cycle.

3. Generally speaking, liquid fabric softeners that you add at the beginning of the final rinse work better than the dryer sheets.
4. Scented baking soda and vinegar are subtle, sweet, natural alternative fabric softeners.
5. *Baking soda and vinegar won't do anything for static cling.* If you find a nontoxic homemade remedy for this, I would love to hear about it. The way I currently avoid static cling is to avoid buying synthetic fabrics. When I do wash synthetics, I either air-dry them or pull them out from the dryer after only a few minutes. You can also try reducing your drying time. Experiment. The attention is worth it. It's overdrying that causes the wear, tear, and aging of your favorites, anyway.

Do You Really Need a Fabric Softener?

If you use only half the amount of detergent you regularly use (as I suggest in my Laundry Detergent section on pp. 191–205), you may find that your clothes naturally feel a lot softer.

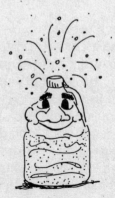

Apple Orchard Laundry Rinse
Fabric Softener

This is my all-time favorite fabric softener. I use apple-scented vinegar a lot in the laundry room. I presoak with it to deodorize and use it in the rinse cycle to soften. It always leaves my laundry with a fresh, clean smell. If you are sensitive to fragrances, try using peppermint-scented vinegar instead.

Ingredients: White distilled vinegar and a fragrance.

How to Make: Add 20 drops of apple fragrance to 1 gallon of white distilled vinegar.

How to Use: Add 1–2 cups vinegar to your rinse cycle as a fabric softener. The vinegar helps to rinse the wash truly clean and dissolve any detergent residue. To deodorize, I add a cup of scented vinegar and presoak for about 30 minutes. Don't add too much vinegar or let it soak too long. Colors will fade with the vinegar (especially inexpensive dyes on rayons). Test a small spot first if you have any doubts.

Effectiveness Rating: 85%

Commercial Brand* vs. Apple Orchard (16-oz. fabric softener): $7.55 vs. $3.60. 1 gallon of vinegar should cost you about $1. The scent will cost about 20¢. I'm estimating 3 gallons of scented vinegar as an equivalent to 16 oz. of Downy. You'll **save** $3.95 each time you refill the bottle.

---

*Price comparison with Downy liquid.

Boing

I developed this recipe for my Bounce-addicted friends. It does nothing to soften or prevent static cling, but it does give your laundry room a sweet scent. Besides, it's just fun to use.

Ingredients: A rag or paper towel and your favorite essential oil.

How to Make: Add 5–10 drops of scent to a rag or paper towel.

What to Do: Scent a rag or paper towel with your favorite laundry scent. Just add a few drops; too much oil could stain your clothes or be a fire hazard. Put the rag in the dryer with your clothes. When I am transferring essential oils from a large bottle to a small bottle, I use a rag to carefully wipe any excess drips of oil. Then I reuse this scented rag in the dryer.

Effectiveness Rating: 30%

Commercial Brand* vs. Boing (16-oz. fabric softener): $2.95 vs. $2.40. The scent should cost you 5¢ a sheet, the paper towel or rag, less than 1¢. Bounce has 40 sheets in a box. You'll **save** 55¢.

---

*Price comparison with Bounce.

Floor Cleaners

What's Really in Them?

Floor cleaners typically contain ammonia, phosphates, detergents, and pine oils. Others contain glycol ethers (like butyl cellosolve), phosphoric acid, potassium hydroxide, and bleach. Floor polishes can contain plastics, glycols, petroleum distillates, petroleum naphtha, nitrobenzene, and ammonia.

What Harm Can They Do?

Floor cleaners can be especially dangerous because they are often left on the floor or under the sink where children can reach them. When swallowed, they can cause nausea, vomiting, stomach pain, bleeding, and/or chemical pneumonia. Cleaners with a high percentage of pine oil in them, such as Pine Sol, are particularly dangerous. If a small child swallows enough of it these cleaners can cause convulsions, coma, and even death. Their strong taste and smell often prevents this from happening, but it can and does happen! Cleaners like Pine Sol are so thin and slippery that they can easily get down a child's air pipe and into the lungs in just the first gulp. The lining of the lungs immediately becomes inflamed and the child tries to unsuccessfully cough it out. In a severe case of chemical pneumonia, the child could be on a respirator in a hospital intensive care unit for a couple of weeks. Later on, the lungs form scar tissue, making it difficult for life for the child to breathe.

Cleaning your floor doesn't have to be dangerous to you and your children. Most people overclean, making more work for themselves or their housekeepers. With a little bit of know-how and a few nontoxic recipes, you can avoid these ridiculously unnecessary problems.

The Three Fantastic Floor-Cleaning Rules

Everybody wants a clean, shiny floor. We are programmed to think that a floor needs to shine for it to be clean. Not so. With modern no-wax and finished floors, we rarely need to polish. In fact, polishing a floor can make it look duller sooner! Here are the facts.

1. *No-wax floor means no need to polish!* Use just a little vinegar or liquid soap and water to clean.
2. Do you have shiny polyurethane-finished wood floors? There's *no need to polish!* A little vinegar or soap and water will clean them just fine.

3. Do you have ceramic tile, brick, or stone floors? There's *no need to polish!* A little vinegar is really all you need to clean.

Polishing a floor when you don't have to do it is a waste of time and money and can make your floor ugly-looking later on. You can clean almost any type of flooring with just a little liquid soap and water and a vinegar rinse. Or just use a little vinegar and baking soda on the spots. Rub soda; dissolve it with the vinegar and the spot is gone. Most of the time, that's all you'll need.

One trick to maintaining a shiny floor is to avoid letting the gritty dirt and grime scratch and dull the surface. Installing good-size mats at every doorway helps. Wiping, cleaning, and/or dust-mopping regularly is important: that's the way to keep a floor shiny and new.

What About Cleaning Wood Floors?

I hate to hear that grit grinding into a wood floor underneath vacuum rollers, so I don't vacuum my wood floors. A good terry cloth dust mop or damp mop works the best. Most of the time you only need to dust-mop with a little of Momma's Earth Mop™ (see pp. 135–36) or my Dust To Dust™ spray (see pp. 146–47) on the mop. If you need more cleaning, you can use a little soap and water. Most wood floors are protected by a varnish, finish, or wax. Only the gentlest of cleaners is required. Many cautious flooring manufacturers recommend only a vinegar-and-water rinse. If you do use vinegar and water, be careful to mop dry the floor after washing. Don't let water spots sit on the floor. Water damages wood and can ruin loose wood tiles, making them buckle and swell. When I clean a wood floor, I throw a dry towel or rag over the loose tiles to protect them from any water overflow and to remind me that they are there.

Many people I know use Murphy's Oil Soap on their wood floors. It cleans well and certainly leaves a nice oily residue. But, remember, even a little bit of oily shine attracts dirt and dust more quickly. A less expensive alternative is to use the ordinary liquid detergent at your kitchen sink. Liquid hand-dishwashing detergents, like Palmolive and Ivory, are gentle and mild cleaners and also make great floor cleaners.

Following are a few of my simple floor-cleaning recipes.

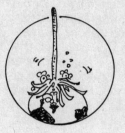

Momma's Earth Mop™
Floor Cleaner

This recipe is a nontoxic cleaning basic. I developed it as a simple floor cleaner, but I found so many uses for its simple scented-vinegar formula that it has found a permanent spot under every sink in my house. It's so easy.

Ingredients: White distilled vinegar, water, and an essential oil for fragrance.

What Else You'll Need: A 16-oz. squirt-bottle.

How to Make: Fill the bottle with equal amounts of white distilled vinegar and water. Add 15–20 drops of pure peppermint oil. Shake to mix.

How to Use: Squirt this refreshing cleaner directly onto the floor and wipe clean with a rag or mop. Use it for linoleum and tile floors in your kitchen, bathroom, and laundry room. It's good for polyurethane and finished wood floors, too. Vinegar is a natural acid that has quick cleaning power and helps to remove the film that typically accumulates on a kitchen floor, but if you have an especially dirty, greasy floor, you may want to use a liquid detergent on it first. Momma's Earth Mop™ is also handy to have in the bathroom because it will cut a light soap film. I use it to eliminate the soap ring in my tub or sink, the film on the shower walls, and the globbies in the soap dish or shower stall. Make sure to get *white* distilled vinegar, not the brown apple cider kind. *Don't forget to add the scent to make this floor cleaner sing.* I like to use a peppermint oil or an apple fragrance. You can purchase both at most natural-food stores or order them by mail from me.

Have fun adding fragrance to your white vinegar. I usually have several scented gallons in my house: one peppermint, one apple, and one tea tree for that medicinal superclean smell. Use about ¼–½ tsp. of fragrance for every gallon of white vinegar. Scented vinegars are great for removing odors left by pet stains, vomit, mildew, sour milk, and more. When we have the flu, I use scented vinegars to get rid of the smell on clothes, sheets, carpet, and floor. Vinegar is reputed to have some germ-killing action.

For extra cleaning power for smudges and scuff marks, sprinkle on a little baking soda (from the shaker on your sink) and rub. Baking soda gets those smudges up fast. Sprinkle on the baking soda, rub, and then squirt on the vinegar for a fast-action fizz that dissolves dirt quickly.

Effectiveness Rating: 90%

Commercial Brand* vs. Momma's Earth Mop™ (32-oz. scented floor cleaner): $6.09 vs. 73¢ 2 cups of vinegar costs 32¢ and the delightful scents cost about 40¢. The purified water costs about 1¢. You'll **save** $5.36 each time you refill the bottle.

*Price comparison with Mop & Glo.

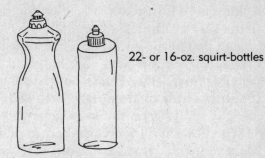

22- or 16-oz. squirt-bottles

How does Momma's Earth Mop™ compare to other commercial floor cleaners and polishes?

When I asked my cleaning-lady friends what it's like to use commercial floor cleaners, here is what they said: "I hate to use them. You put them on and the dirt builds up, and then you have to use ammonia and hot water to get it off. The [floor] edges are always really dirty. It makes you do twice the work. Put it on and take it off, only to put it on again. We usually tell all our clients it's a waste of time to use it. Vinegar and water makes the floor shine just fine."

People put on the Mop & Glo. It makes the floor dull, and then they ask us to clean it, and then they ask us to put it on again! I just hate the bottle, the whole thing. We tell people it just isn't good for the floor. It makes you do things twice, *but some people don't seem to care.*

What about using Mr. Clean?

The scented vinegar and water is so much easier to use. You just squirt it on and wipe it up with a towel. With Mr. Clean, you have to get a bucket and mix it. Then you have to soap the floor and rinse it. It never really rinses well and leaves the floor sticky. You can feel it under your shoes. We use the vinegar and water for ceramic and tile floors especially. It really makes them shine.

- Momma's Earth Mop™ is great for cleaning tubs and the soapy film in shower stalls. I have a small plastic sink that fits over the bathtub for my little daughter to use. She loves to wash her hands in it. The sink gets very slimy. After I dump out the slimy soapy water, I squirt a little of Momma's Earth Mop, which cleans it right up. It's great for soap dishes, too.
- When I want a superclean bathroom floor, I use Merlin's Magic™, my tea tree oil, soap, and water recipe (see p. 114), in a spray- or squirt-bottle, then follow up with a rinse of vinegar. It's important to rinse with that vinegar so that the floor isn't slippery or sticky from leftover soap film.

To many cleaning professionals, the idea of using white distilled vinegar to clean floors is no surprise. What does surprise them is the idea of scenting the vinegar. Vinegar all by itself smells really pungent. If you are the type who complains whenever your mother uses vinegar to clean the floor, then get her a present. Pick up a bottle of peppermint oil and drop some in her vinegar before she cleans. You'll both notice the blissful difference.

Home Chemistry: Lesson 1. Vinegar vs. Grease

I've read that vinegar cuts grease in so many reference books that I thought it was true. I finally put vinegar to the test. I dipped my hands in a greasy pan and tried to wash off the grease with the vinegar. Still greasy. Next I tried baking soda. It worked okay, but not great. Then I tried the liquid detergent at my sink. The detergent took the grease off best but left a sticky residue on my fingers that took a lot of water to rinse off.

I had several other people do the same experiment. Their results were the same. *Vinegar does not cut grease.* That makes sense because vinegar and oils are both acidic, so they don't neutralize each other. Perhaps vinegar got the reputation for cutting grease on floors because it was cutting that ugly soap and detergent residue. A sticky detergent film collects dust and grease, particularly in the kitchen.

Home Chemistry: Lesson 2. Vinegar vs. Mineral Deposits

Soap and baking soda are alkaline and therefore neutralize and clean up acidic dirt and oils. Mineral deposits are alkaline, and acids such as vinegar work to neutralize and dissolve them. That's why vinegar is suggested for water deposits. Generally speaking, vinegar is much too mild of an acid to be of real help in dissolving a significant mineral deposit. But it can work to prevent deposits from building up.

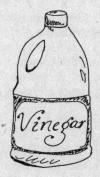

Dishy-Wishy Floor Cleaner

Floor Cleaner

What's the least expensive way to clean your floors? Use a squirt or two of hand-dishwashing liquid in a bucket, a sponge or rag mop, and you're done.

Ingredient: Liquid soap or detergent, water, and perhaps a scented vinegar rinse.

What Else You'll Need: A bucket, a mop, and/or rags and towels.

How to Make: Use only 1 or 2 squirts for a full bucket of water—more if you use a liquid soap, less if you use a detergent.

How to Use: Hand-dishwashing liquid detergents are great all-purpose cleaners, but you don't need much, so don't be too eager with that squirting. Use too much and you will leave a soapy film to which tomorrow's dirt will cling. Sometimes I use a scented vinegar rinse to make sure that every bit of that soap or detergent is gone. And the scented vinegars can make the whole kitchen smell good. Use a good-size squirt-bottle to apply the rinse, then dry with towels or terry-cloth mop. For this recipe, I like to use Dr. Bronner's liquid soap instead of the detergent because it rinses off easily and smells good right from the start.

Effectiveness Rating: 100%

Commercial Brand* vs. Dishy-Wishy Floor Cleaner (20-oz. floor cleaner): $2.59 vs. 40¢. The dishwashing detergent costs less than 1¢ a squirt! About 40¢ worth of dishwashing liquid makes about 40 gallons. You'll **save** $2.19 each time you refill the bottle.

---

*Price comparison with Mr. Clean.

Forest Floor

This recipe is for you Pine Sol–aholics. Pine Sol smells great but can be dangerous to have around the house. These non-toxic alternatives are safe and smell even better.

Ingredients: Dr. Bronner's Sal Suds.

How to Make: Use 2 or 3 good squirts (or 2 to 3 tbsp.) of Sal Suds in a bucket.

How to Use: Many of us are addicted to the pine scent in Pine Sol. Scents create strong associations; we've grown up thinking that if it smells like pine, then it must be clean. That scent keeps us hooked on toxic cleaners. Fortunately for us, Jim Bronner, Dr. Bronner's son, took the time to develop the perfect environmentally safer substitute for Pine Sol. "Sal Suds is about as natural as you can make a powerful cleaner," says Jim, now president of the company. The pine scent you get from Sal Suds is much more refined and sweet. "It's the highest quality pine oil we can get," says Jim. You can truly smell the difference.

Effectiveness Rating: 100%

Why Isn't the Pine Oil in Sal Suds Toxic Like the Pine Oil in Pine Sol?

Pine Sol contains 20% pine oil, giving it properties that make it quite toxic to ingest. Sal Suds contains less than 1% pine needle oil, used primarily as a fragrance.

Do You Have a Shiny New Floor?

Ordinary household dirt underneath your shoes acts like sandpaper on a shiny floor, dulling it and ruining that bright, shiny gloss. To make life easier, add several feet of high-quality mats to all your entrances, and you'll track in less dirt and have to sweep less. You can get professional-quality mats from several of the catalogs I've listed in the Resources section (see pp. 283–89). Mats are important. Dirt on your shoes wears down your carpets as well. Invest in these cleaning time savers! In our house, sandy or especially dirty shoes and socks are taken off at the front door so that scratchy dirt stays there.

Do Your Floors Look Dull and Grimy?

Dull, grimy floors may be that way because they have a leftover detergent residue. Try using a scented vinegar to rinse it away. On the other hand, the floor may just be old and the finish has been worn away.

What Can Be Done with a Worn and Scratched Vinyl Floor?

A polish will coat your floor in a thin layer of plastic and may help your floor to look better temporarily, but it will soon dull again. Instead of spending your money on a polish for a temporary fix, it makes more sense to save your "cleaning" money for a new floor. You can also try applying a paste wax just in the areas that need it.

It's tempting to want to make that floor shine. Don't make the mistake that I did. . . . I had just finished cleaning a lovely wood floor and I thought it was time for a polish. It didn't need it, but I just thought it would look nice. So I grabbed my It's A Lotsa Polish™ furniture polish and started squirting. I rubbed it in. It looked nice at first, but it was oily and sticky and I started tracking the oil onto the carpet—big mistake. Of course, the wood floor had a nice plastic-type finish on it, and the oil just sat on top of it looking shiny, slimy and collecting dirt. It was another 30 minutes or so before I finished washing that floor down with soap and water again to clean off that oil. Most modern wood floors and furniture have a nice finish on them to protect them from water damage. Putting an oily polish on them to make them shine only makes them oily.

Cleaning a Floor with Years of Dirt on It?

You don't really need anything fancy to clean a tough job—you certainly don't need expensive, toxic chemicals. It's the motivation and mojo that counts. I've cleaned layers of dirt off kitchen and linoleum floors by scrubbing with just my Earth Scrub™ (baking soda and liquid soap recipe; see pp. 239–40) and a sturdy toilet brush.

1. Squirt on the Earth Scrub™. Scrub the floor thoroughly with a high-quality toilet bowl brush or professional long-handled scrubber. Don't use a toilet brush with a metal wire center. Those things don't work very well, are a waste of money, and worst of all, they *scratch*. Throw them away. Next time, buy the more expensive kind with the sturdy plastic center.
2. Let the scrub soak in for a bit before you start scrubbing again, and the dirt will literally lift off.
3. Dry-wipe with old towels or rags. A dry-wipe picks up most of the now dirty baking soda and soap on the floor. This saves you water and rinsing time. Toss the towels in for laundering with your other cleaning rags.
4. Squirt on plenty of scented vinegar rinse. Mop dry with more old towels. I walk around on the towels so I don't have to bend over. Squirt again, and towel-dry some more. The feet-on-towels method is pretty effective, and it's a fun break after all that scrubbing. Make sure to use plenty of scented vinegar rinse to get the soap–and–baking soda residue thoroughly washed off.

◆

Furniture Polishes

What's Really in Them?

Furniture polishes can contain a wide range of nasty chemicals: petroleum distillates, nitrobenzenes, phenols, pine oil, alcohol, waxes, acetate, turpentine, shellac, silicones, mineral spirits, ammonia, and formaldehyde. The spray types can contain waxes, silicone oils, mineral oils, naphthas, perfumes, formaldehyde, and propellants.

What Harm Can They Do?

One of the most hazardous thing about furniture polishes is that they can be appealing to small children to drink. To a small child, colored polishes can look dangerously like a fruit drink; others can look like milk. Lemon-oil furniture polishes can not only look and smell like a tasty lemon drink but be lemon flavored, too. If your child has swallowed any, call the Poison Control Center right away. Some of those polishes can easily slip down a child's air pipe and into the lungs to cause chemical pneumonia. Chemical pneumonia can cause scarring of the lung tissue that could give a child a medical condition similar to the emphysema of a smoker of 20 or 30 years.

Furniture polishes are particularly dangerous because people don't consider them to be dangerous. Everybody knows how dangerous drain cleaners are, but if you ask someone if furniture polishes are dangerous, you'll often get "I don't know" for an answer. And if you look under the kitchen sink, you'll often find those furniture polishes right where curious little hands can get at them.

Since 1989, some polishes have changed formulations

to be less risky, but others have not. Why risk it when you can make your own—even edible—alternatives?

Many furniture polishes also contain chemicals federally classified as hazardous, such as petroleum distillates, phenol, and nitrobenzene, which technically makes them hazardous waste—expensive waste for your city to deal with and potentially environmentally damaging.

What About the Spray-Type Furniture Polishes?

Personally, I just don't like the smells or the sprays, and the aerosols are such a waste. I can't count how many cans of Endust and Pledge I have seen in wastebaskets. But that's also because *there is so little cleaner in them!* Your typical furniture polish spray can cost you over $4 and has only 10 oz. of cleaner in it. And as I'm sure you've experienced, 10 oz. doesn't go very far when you are dusting and cleaning the house. Also, please don't fall for the "an aerosol can is steel and can be recycled" argument. Refilling your plastic spray-bottle with your own homemade formula is by far the most environmentally kind choice. The propellants, expensive manufacturing process, and lack of recycling programs make aerosol cans an environmental loser.

Should You Use an Oily Furniture Polish or a Spray Type?

There are two different types of furniture polish that you should be aware of: the spray-on dust-and-clean kind and the oily kind. *Today, most furniture is finished with varnishes and plastics, so it hardly needs any oil at all.* Not only is using an oily furniture polish on a finished piece of furniture unnecessary, but the oil makes it sticky enough to collect dust and dirt all the more rapidly. On the other hand, unfinished or lightly finished wood needs the conditioning and protection of a natural oil. So, I've developed two different recipes for you. The first is the dust-and-clean kind, called Dust To Dust™. The second is an oily type called It's A Lotsa Polish™. For the varnished wood furniture, cupboards, and bookshelves I use the Dust To Dust™. On unfinished and lightly finished wood furniture, such as my oak coffee table and entertainment center, I use It's A Lotsa Polish™. According to my test results, both of these formulas perform equally as well as—if not better than—most commercial products.

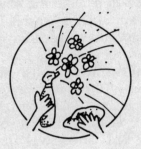

Dust to Dust™

Furniture Polish

This is as effective as any store-bought product! You'll love this formula because it works so well, smells great, and at 30¢ a bottle, the price can't be beaten!

Ingredients: Olive oil (preferably the light kind), white distilled vinegar, pure essential lemon oil (or lemon juice), and water.

What Else You'll Need: A 16-oz. spray-bottle.

How to Make: Put 2 tsp. olive oil in the bottle. Add 20 drops or more of pure essential lemon oil. Add ¼ cup of white distilled vinegar. Fill the rest of the bottle with water (purified is best). Shake well. *Be sure to use a pure essential lemon oil, not the chemical synthetics.* You can use fresh lemon juice instead of the lemon oil. I usually don't suggest this because the juice will spoil in the bottle if not refrigerated. If you use up most or all of the cleaner fairly quickly, then lemon juice is a nice substitute for the lemon oil. Use 1–2 tsp. juice in place of the 20 drops of oil. Make sure to strain the juice well or the pulp will clog the squirter. If you don't have a strainer, try using a coffee filter.

How to Use: Spray this formula on your rag or directly onto furniture. Wipe it dry immediately. It's great for the weekly dusting and cleaning of the wood in your house. I've used this formula on cabinets, furniture, wood paneling, and picture frames. The olive oil conditions and the vinegar cleans. For wood that is drying out from age or water exposure (a typical place for white, dried-out wood areas are the cabinets underneath any sink), add more olive oil to the recipe or condition them first with my It's A Lotsa Polish™ recipe (see pp. 149–50).

You can use Dust To Dust™ for your dust-mopping, too. A couple of good squirts on your dust mop will help to pick up dust quickly on any hardwood floor. I've also used it to clean spills off leather coaches and even my leather jacket—works great and costs pennies. The vinegar and olive oil will separate in this formula, so *shake well before each use*.

Effectiveness Rating: 90%–100%

Commercial Brand* vs. Dust To Dust™ (10-oz. furniture polish spray): $4.73 vs. 60¢. 2 tsp. olive oil costs 26¢, ¼ cup of vinegar, only 4¢. The refreshing lemon scent should cost you about 30¢. You'll **save** $4.13 each time you refill the bottle.

---

*Price comparison with Endust.

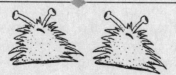

To Dust or Not to Dust, That Is the Question

I never thought it was important to dust until I found out what is *in* dust. Dust mites love to feed on the things you can find in dust, such as bits of skin, hair, and food.

I don't know if I'm allergic to mites, but I know I don't like the idea of having them around. Dust has suspicious stuff in it: mites—both dead and alive—and mite parts, pet and people hair and skin flakes, lint, insect parts, disintegrated stuffing, foam and fabric bits, powdered detergents, bacteria, road dust, bits of tires, tar, pesticides, fertilizers, oils, particles from industry emissions, ash from incinerators and fires, flying garbage truck debris . . . yuck! Let's get rid of the dust.

I've bought fancy microcloths to dust with, but I can never find them when I need them. Your basic slightly damp, soft cotton cloth works great. Dust To Dust™ formula is a great substitute for something like Pledge or Endust.

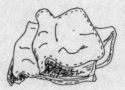

THE SEARCH FOR GOLD DUST

There are two ways to dust: you can be repelled by the really dusty places and try to avoid them or you can consider dusting to be like a search for gold dust. My favorite dirty places to find "gold" dust are on top of the refrigerator, window and door sills, light bulbs, picture frames, plants, and on top of the computer, fax, and answering machines. Dust also loves to collect in the lower regions of your house, like the bottom bookshelves and the legs and rungs of furniture. Other assorted items that live on the floor, such as printers, books, and animal cages, are all great dust caches. The dirtier your rag, the healthier you are.

Now, here's something to polish your furniture with.

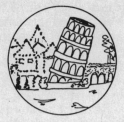

It's A Lotsa Polish™

Furniture Polish

I love this furniture polish because it is gentle to use: no sprays, strange odors, metal cans, and no irritating chemicals. Best of all, this formula is absolutely edible: wipe on furniture—or sprinkle on salad or pasta!

Ingredients: Olive oil, white distilled vinegar, and food-grade pure essential lemon oil or lemon juice.

What Else You'll Need: A small 8-oz. squirt-bottle.

8-oz. flip-top bottle

How to Make: Add ¾ cup olive oil to the bottle, then add ¼ cup white distilled vinegar. To save time, I usually estimate this recipe by filling the bottle ¾ full of olive oil and then filling to the top with vinegar. Add the vinegar slowly because it's easy to pour in too much and overflow. For fragrance, add 50 drops or ¼ tsp. of lemon oil last. You don't have to include the lemon oil if you don't have it on hand; the nutty smell of vinegar, oil, and wood is nice all by itself. By the way, using a funnel for this recipe can make the whole thing neater. *Be sure to use a pure essential lemon oil, not the chemical synthetics*. As with the Dust To Dust™ recipe, you can use fresh lemon juice instead of the lemon oil (see that recipe—on pp. 146–47—for the instructions). If you don't have any lemon oil, you can also try scenting it with a ½ tsp. or so of vanilla extract instead.

How to Use: Squirt this polish onto a terry cloth rag or directly on furniture. I have used this formula on oak, maple, cherry, mahogany, and teak with great results. The olive oil nourishes the wood as well as making it beautiful. Use more vinegar if your furniture is really dirty, or less if you want just a nice shine. Vinegar can also help to remove any water marks; but be careful, because too much vinegar can damage the finish. Test your formula first on a furniture leg or side. Cup your hand when you squirt the polish onto the rag, and you'll give the polish some time to soak in. Otherwise, the polish can roll right off and onto your clothes, sofa, or rug. When I can, I also squirt the polish directly onto the furniture itself and then rub it in. *Shake well before each use.*

Effectiveness Rating: 90%–100%

Commercial Brand* vs. It's A Lotsa Polish™ (16-oz. oil-based furniture polish): $4.39 vs. $2.60. 1 1/2 cups olive oil costs $2.32; 1/2 cup vinegar costs 8¢. The refreshing lemon scent should cost you about 20¢. You'll **save** $1.79 each time you refill the bottle.

*Price comparison with Old English.

Here are some tips for using It's A Lotsa Polish™:

- Both wood and leather have natural oils in them that evaporate over time. It is important to restore these natural oils to maintain the longevity and health of your furniture and leather items. Many furniture polishes just use plastics to make furniture shiny.
- It does matter what kind of oil you use. Walnut oil or linseed oil are excellent alternatives to the olive oil, but they are more expensive. You can usually get walnut or linseed oil at your local hardware store. If you're on a budget and if you can't afford the olive oil, you can substitute a vegetable oil instead.
- Remember to be careful with the amount of vinegar. Vinegar is a mild acid, and too much vinegar can damage a finish. If you have a beautiful piece of wood

furniture and you would scream if you were to ruin it, then make sure to test your formula on the furniture's leg or an underneath piece first.

If you'd like to introduce nontoxic cleaning alternatives to a friend, try demonstrating with this formula. Most people have the olive oil and vinegar in their house and are happy to have you volunteer to polish their furniture. The recipe is also easy to remember: 3 parts olive oil to 1 part vinegar. Never underestimate the power of a simple idea.

THE CHICKEN-OR-THE-EGG PROBLEM: SHOULD I VACUUM OR DUST FIRST?

Yes, most vacuums can blow dust around your house. The chicken: if you dust first, then the dust you wipe off your shelves goes onto the floor, where you then attempt to vacuum it up, but in the process, you blow dust all over the house again, and then you need to dust again! The egg: if you vacuum first and then dust, the dust you wipe off your shelves goes onto the floor, and then you need to vacuum again! It's a ridiculous problem but fun to think about. I always dust after I vacuum because the dust I capture usually stays stuck to my rag.

WHY DON'T YOU LIKE TO VACUUM?

Vacuums can certainly blow dust around your house, especially if the bag is full. I noticed that my nose and I were always a little stuffy and irritated after vacuuming. Vacuums also don't work very well when the bag is full. *I've read that when a vacuum bag is only half full, the vacuum is actually 50% less efficient.* Wow. For a quick vacuum-dust prevention technique, I spray water on the outside of the bag before I vacuum, and I keep spraying as I vacuum. Spraying water works fairly well, but it is kind of annoying to do. If you have a real dust allergy, it's better to get the canister kind of vacuum with long attachments and leave the canister outside the room while you vacuum. Using an inexpensive dust mask works fairly well, too.

Lotsa Leather

This is another version of the It's A Lotsa Polish™ recipe, but it's for cleaning leather. I've used this recipe for my leather car seat, boots, and jackets. It cleans and conditions beautifully without adding the toxic chemical smell that most commercial leather cleaners do.

Ingredients: Olive oil and white distilled vinegar.

What Else You'll Need: A small 8-oz. squirt-bottle.

How to Make: The ratio is 2 parts olive oil to 1 part vinegar. For an 8-oz. bottle, use ⅔ cup of olive oil and ⅓ cup of vinegar. Or just fill any size bottle approximately ⅔ full of olive oil and the remaining ⅓ with vinegar.

How to Use: Clean and condition your leather couches, purses, car seats, jackets, and even your leather boots with this easy formula. Shake well, squirt, and rub in. I usually use my It's A Lotsa Polish™ bottle but add just a little more vinegar. Don't squirt on too much, or it will leave the leather sticky. Buff dry with a soft cloth. *Don't use this formula on suede.* For spots on suede, try rubbing gently with a fine-grade sandpaper or hard-bristle brush. If you use the oil on suede, you'll really get a stain! *Shake well before using*.

Effectiveness Rating: 70%

Glass Cleaners

What's Really in Them?

Glass cleaners usually contain ammonia, alcohol, butyl cellosolve, detergents, silicone, waxes, formaldehyde, and lots of water. More so than any other cleaner, when you buy a glass cleaner, you are paying a *premium* price for mostly just *plain water*.

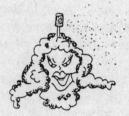

What Harm Can They Do?

Even though most glass cleaners contain only a trace of ammonia, it can be irritating to the respiratory tract. Ammonia should be especially avoided if you or your children have such respiratory problems as asthma or bronchitis. What you really don't want to do is to try making your own glass cleaner with ammonia and make it much too strong! *Small children, older people, and those with even mild respiratory problems are better off not breathing any ammonia.* The problem is that when cleaning glass, we usually spray a fine mist of ammonia, detergents, and other chemicals and then lean right into it and breathe deeply while wiping the glass vigorously. I haven't figured out a way to use a glass cleaner without simply inhaling it. If you are a cleaning professional, then you probably worry that years of constant use and inhaling cleaning chemicals like this might contribute to chemical sensitivities. The smell simply irritates me, so I try to avoid it. Ammonia is a poison when ingested and is particularly dangerous when combined with other cleaners that contain bleach, thus creating toxic chloramine gas.

So, You Want Perfect Windows, Do You?

Very few cleaning chores inspire our desire for perfection as much as windows do. The fact is that most commercial glass cleaners perform poorly and unreliably. Consumer Reports Books says, "Many of the glass cleaners on the market are mediocre products. Homemade recipes can equal or best many of the aerosols, sprays, and premoistened towels in the stores."* Streaking can be a problem with any glass cleaner. The way to avoid streaking is to dry the glass completely: keep wiping until it's dry. Washing windows in the hot sun causes streaks because the cleaner dries before you get a chance to wipe it off.

The Search for the Perfect Glass Cleaner

In retrospect, I think it would have been easier to find the Holy Grail than to find the perfect nontoxic glass cleaner. My assistant, Bonnie, and I spent days and days in frustration, trying out all the recipes in the books—cornstarch, vinegar, soap and vinegar, washing soda, even salty water! The cornstarch solutions worked well but clogged the sprayer; the vinegar solutions worked inside the house but streaked and spotted the car windows;

---

*Florman, Monte, and Marjorie Florman. *How to Clean Practically Anything*, p. 64. New York: Consumer Reports Books (a division of Consumers Union), 1993.

the soap and vinegar solutions left the predictable ugly soap film. Nothing worked like we wanted it to. I kept grabbing for that smelly blue commercial stuff to use as a comparison to our formulas. The commercial stuff didn't work all the time, either!

Why not try a little club soda? I thought. *The books say it shines floors.* The club soda turned out to work just great. The big test came when I tried it out on two housekeepers. One of the ladies simply asked for the regular glass cleaner. I handed her a spray-bottle of club soda instead. Fifteen minutes later, I wandered in and asked her how it had worked. She just smiled and nodded. The mirrors were sparkly clean. A couple of weeks later, I had another lady in to help me out with my new baby. She offered to do some cleaning as well. I handed her my homemade floor cleaner, tub and tile cleaner, and glass cleaner. I returned an hour later. The bathroom was sparkling and so was she. "I really liked that glass cleaner," she said. "It's great." She grinned. "It really leaves a sparkle and it doesn't smell. The other cleaners always make me sneeze." *Ahhhh . . . what a discovery,* I thought.

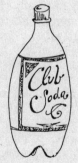

Do We Really Need to Clean Our Windows with Something Blue?

Why do we insist on making life more complicated than it is? What could be simpler than club soda? One

Club Clean™
Glass Cleaner

This is one of my best recipes: plain club soda as a window cleaner—easy, inexpensive, and effective. You will be amazed at how great it works, and at a little more than a penny an ounce, it's a bargain compared to any commercial cleaner!

Ingredients: Club soda (found in the soda section of your grocery store).

What Else You'll Need: An 8- or 16-oz. spray-bottle.

How to Make: Fill the bottle with plain club soda.

How to Use: Spray and wipe. All glass cleaners work best with a lint-free cloth. I find that a soft cotton terry-cloth rag works best. I use Club Clean™ for my mirrors, windows, glass tables, eyeglasses, even the photocopy machine. For the absolutely best results, use two lint-free rags: one rag for the first wet-wipe and one for the dry-wipe. This method eliminates the streaking that comes from using a dirty, wet rag. Club soda doesn't dry as quickly as commercial cleaners, but I guarantee you that when it dries, the glass will be sparkling clean. What's the magic ingredient? Sodium citrate. The sodium citrate softens the water and helps to clean. My neighbor says it works better than most commercial brands. If your windows are extra dirty, wet your rag with the club soda, add a teeny-tiny sprinkle of baking soda or an itsy-bitsy squirt of hand-dish-washing liquid, then wet your rag again. Rub the glass, spray well, and wipe: the grime is gone. Professional cleaners love this glass cleaner that has no nasty ammonia smell.

Effectiveness Rating: 95%

Commercial Brand* vs. Club Clean™ (22-oz. glass cleaner): $2.69 vs. 31¢. Club soda costs only 1 1/2¢ an ounce! You'll **save** $2.38 each time you refill the bottle.

---

*Price comparison with Windex.

of my cleaning-lady friends loved it so much that she "sneaks" it into her client's house. She cleans a lot of houses and breathes a lot of ammonia. What a relief to have an alternative to that irritating ammonia smell. If you must clean with something blue, try adding a drop of blue food coloring to your cleaner. Tests have shown that people think a glass cleaner works better if it's blue!

Club Clean™ Comes in Handy for Other Uses, Too

STAIN MASTER I

It's handy to have a bottle of club soda around when you get a nasty stain on your shirt, tie, dress, or table-cloth. A couple of good squirts and a rub with a hand-dishwashing liquid (quick, quick, quick, let it sit, then rinse) will handle many everyday stains.

STAIN MASTER II

I've also used club soda for nasty carpet spills like wine, juice, or tomato sauce. With a paper towel, try to blot up as much of the spill as you can as quickly as possible, working from outside in. Next, use an old towel and step on it to get what had soaked into the padding. Now, give it a quick pour of club soda—not too much, or you will spread the stain. Blot again. Next, try using a little spray of soap and water to finish picking up the rest of the stain.

IT'S A LEAF DUSTER!

While washing my windows, I also use Club Clean™ to clean my plants. I spray the plant all over and then gently wipe the dust and dirt off the leaves. Plants grow better without the dust clogging up their leaves. It's very handy to use, and the plants love it.

SHINE THE CHROME IN YOUR HOME

Use Club Clean™ to shine the chrome fixtures in your bathroom and kitchen, too. Add a drop or two of oil to your rag and they'll really shine and prevent water spots from collecting. Simply beautiful.

If you run out of club soda, use purified water instead. Amazingly enough, Consumer Reports Books rated plain water as a glass cleaner at the top of their list in effectiveness and price.* I've found that using purified water is even better.

Isn't Using Newspapers a Good Way to Clean Windows and Recycle the Papers at the Same Time?

Newspapers clean windows because of the solvent power of the inks used in them. When you clean with them, you expose yourself to the smells and residues of those toxic inks. Chemically sensitive people will tell you there is no way they would clean with them. Also, when you clean windows with a newspaper, the inks get all over your hands—sometimes on the window sills, and the paper wads up into a big soggy mess that usually doesn't go into your newspaper recycling bin. Cleaning with a little soapy water and a towel is much more pleasant, to say the least.

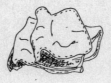

---

*Florman, Monte, and Marjorie Florman. *How to Clean Practically Anything.* p. 66. New York: Consumer Reports Books (a division of Consumers Union), 1993.

Dishy-Wishy Window Washer
Outdoor Window Cleaner

What's the best way to wash those outdoor windows? Everybody has a favorite. Using the liquid hand-dishwashing detergent at your sink is one of the cheapest and easiest products with which to wash your outside windows. Here is my professional-tested, time-tested, and inexpensive recipe.

Ingredients: Any liquid detergent, water, and perhaps some white distilled vinegar.

What Else You'll Need: A bucket, sponges, a squeegee, and drying rags or towels.

How to Make: You need only 1 squirt of liquid detergent for a full bucket of water.

How to Use: Any liquid detergent works great as an outdoor window cleaner because it lubricates your squeegee and helps to get off the tougher kind of outdoor dust, dirt, and grime that accumulates on windows. Don't use *too much* detergent or you will get streaks and hazy windows from the leftover film. If you do get a film, you can take care of it quickly and easily with a vinegar rinse. To apply the vinegar rinse, use a sprayer, squirt-bottle, or sponge—whatever is easiest and most suited to the job. I like to use a vinegar rinse anyway because it makes the windows squeaky clean. If you are a window-washing perfectionist, you'll want to use purified water in your bucket, too.

Effectiveness Rating: 100%

Commercial Brand* vs. Dishy-Wishy Window Washer (22-oz. glass cleaner): $2.69 vs. 2¢. The dishwashing detergent costs less than 1¢ a squirt! You'll **save** $2.67.

---

*Price comparison with Windex.

Here's my favorite outdoor window-cleaning method:

1. *First, put one squirt of liquid soap or hand-dishwashing detergent in a bucket of warm water.* If I have several windows to do, I like to prepare at least two buckets ahead of time. I also set out several clean old terry washcloths or towels for drying and a sponge, rag, or window wand for the washing. Don't forget the squeegee! It's possible to do big windows without it but a squeegee makes it much easier. *For hard water areas:* this may seem like a silly suggestion, but if you have a home purifier and you want superclean windows, use the purified water. Minerals get in the way of any cleaning, and the minerals in the water will stand out like sore spots when you are washing windows. A vinegar rinse will help get those spots off, too.

2. *Next, grab your rag or sponge and wash the sills first* and rinse so that none of that creepy black sill dirt comes slithering down the windows after they are cleaned. If your window sills are very dirty, you will want to soap them all up and spray them off with a garden hose before you even attempt to start on the windows.

3. *Once the sills are clean, I start on the windows. Soap up those windows with a sponge or rag and get at any dirty or crusty spots.* Use a putty knife or razor blade set to scrape off the stuck-ons. I always use the razor blade wet and push forward on it—never back and forth, which could permanently scratch the window.

4. *Once all the grime is loosened and soaped, use the squeegee.* Work from top to bottom. Keep that squeegee blade clean but wet for a nice, even wipe. I like to follow up closely behind my squeegee with a vinegar rinse. As I squeeze on the vinegar and watch the soap film dissolve, I finish with the second squeegee wipe.

The vinegar rinse isn't necessary, but the perfectionist in me likes it. If I have a lot of windows to do, I skip the rinse. When and where necessary, I dry the windows with an old terry cloth towel. I'm especially careful to dry drippy edges of the windows and window sills before they muddy up something else.

5. *Refill the squirt-bottle with vinegar and start soaping up another window.* Washing windows outside is a refreshing kind of exercise best done on a cool but sunny day. Although it may seem appealing, it's aggravating to wash windows on a very hot, sunny day, because your windows will dry before you get a chance to wipe them and you will end up with streaks. If you are going to wash windows on a hot day, start with the shady side of the house first and let the sun go down a little before you get to the sunny side.

6. *Get someone to pay you money for washing the windows, even if it's just a quarter.* You deserve a little reward for making the world a cleaner place. I started washing windows for my mom for a couple of dollars when I was 10. I loved earning the money and enjoyed the challenge of getting them clean.

"I Tried Your Nontoxic Glass Cleaners and My Windows Came Out Looking Muddy. What's Wrong?"

If you cleaned your windows the nontoxic way, but they still look dirty, it's possible that commercial cleaners have left a waxy coating on your windows—and mirrors. Clean surfaces first with a liquid soap and water, and then follow with a good rinse of vinegar. If they are really muddy, try using a bit of baking soda on your rag as a scrub. A good rinse with vinegar will take away any baking-soda residue. Now you're ready to enjoy the nontoxic alternatives.

Paint Spray in Your View?

I had some windows with corners that were covered with a fine mist of paint spots. Here's what I did to get rid of most of them.

Ingredients: Baking soda and white distilled vinegar.

What Else You'll Need: A white nylon-backed sponge.

How to Use: It takes a razor blade to get off most paint spots. But what about those annoying tiny paint spots? If your windows just seem rough when you run the squeegee across them, you may have a fine mist of paint spray on them. To get those tiny paint spots off, I use a little nontoxic baking soda and a white nylon-backed sponge instead of having to get out that dangerous razor blade set. Put the soda on your sponge and rub. Use the back of the sponge to get at the more tenacious spots. The baking soda takes off 50% of the spots and makes the whole window easier to clean. To finish, dissolve that baking-soda residue with a lovely scented vinegar rinse, and you'll have a new outlook on life.

Effectiveness Rating: 50%

Window Dressing
Glass Cleaner

When I run out of club soda, I use this recipe. I call it Window Dressing because it reminds me to clean those ever-toothpaste-spotted bathroom mirrors at the same time as I'm getting dressed.

Ingredients: White distilled vinegar, water, and perhaps, an essential oil.

What Else You'll Need: An 8- or 16-oz. clean spray-bottle.

How to Make: Fill a spray-bottle half with vinegar and half with water. You can add a few drops of lemon or peppermint oil (up to 8 drops) to mask the vinegar smell if you like.

How to Use: Vinegar and water is a very popular homemade glass-cleaner, but I don't like the smell of *plain* vinegar in a small enclosed space like a bathroom. Adding a lemon or peppermint scent helps and doesn't seem to dull the cleaning. Occasionally, I'll use my Nature Made™ vinegar air freshener formula (see p. 71) that's already on the bathroom counter as a quick and handy glass cleaner. This formula works well but doesn't dry as quickly as the club soda. Be sure to wipe completely dry.

Effectiveness Rating: 80%

Lemon Aid for Windows
Glass Cleaner

This is a great grease-cutting and fresh-smelling glass cleaner, especially if you use fresh lemons. Add a little more lemon juice and some liquid soap and you've got a great all-purpose kitchen cleaner, too.

Ingredients: Lemon juice and purified water.

What Else You'll Need: A 16-oz. spray-bottle and a fine-mesh strainer (like an old-style tea strainer).

How to Make: Add 1–2 tsp. lemon juice to 16 oz. water. Make sure to strain the lemon juice before adding.

How to Use: This cleaner works great for particularly dirty or greasy windows like the sliding glass door area where the kids' hand- and noseprints are gathered and the place the dog likes to slobber on as part of his begging technique. Fresh lemon juice works best, but be sure to strain it well. If you don't have a fine-mesh strainer, you can squeeze the lemon juice through a coffee filter. I've also used the store-bought reconstituted lemon juice, but it's not as effective. Using purified water definitely improves performance. Lemon juice will spoil, so use up the entire bottle or refrigerate after use.

Effectiveness Rating: 90%

A note on my glass cleaner ratings: I rated my club soda recipe better than Lemon Aid for Windows for a couple of reasons. The Lemon Aid doesn't dry as quickly as the club soda and has a tendency to leave residual spray marks. It also takes more time to make than simply filling a spray-bottle with club soda. The most compelling reason of all is that because Lemon Aid has lemon juice in it, it needs to be refrigerated if you plan on leaving it in the bottle very long. I don't want to have to refrigerate my glass cleaner, so it's club soda for me!

Insecticides and Other Pest Controls

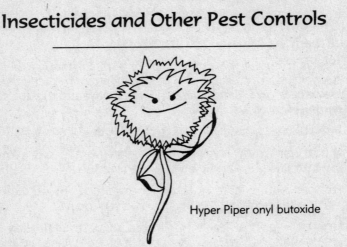

Hyper Piper onyl butoxide

This section of the book is for those of you looking for nontoxic or least-toxic alternatives to some of the nastier chemicals we have around the house to control insects and other small nuisances. Keeping your house free of insects and uninvited small animals is an important part of keeping your house clean. I haven't covered every kind of pest control, but I've included five of the most popular ones: ants, cockroaches, fleas, mice, and plant pests.

What's Really in Them?

The spray type of insecticides for ants and roaches can contain synthetic pyrethrins, rotenone, piperonyl butoxide, and tetramethrin. Other insecticides can contain nicotine, copper naphthenate, and petroleum derivatives. The more toxic include chlordane, dichlorobenzene, and organophosphates such as the parathions.

What Harm Can They Do?

Most people are aware of the dangers of insecticides and other pest controls and don't want to use them, but they don't want the pests, either. I've tried to find the very best of the easy and least-toxic solutions for you that really work. Don't expect miracles, and don't go for the "kill them all" mentality. We do live on the planet with other creatures, and they deserve our respect and love, too.

Beware of old insecticides! Many contain highly toxic ingredients like arsenic, dichlorodiphenyltrichloroethane (DDT), lead, and copper. Old insecticides should never be used, and they should never be thrown into the garbage. It may be a hassle, but they need to be responsibly brought to a hazardous-waste disposal center. If we want to speak the truth here, *they should never have been put on the market in the first place.*

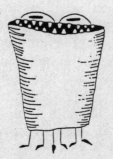

We are in no safer a position today. The screening process for introducing a new chemical in home products sold in the marketplace is severely inadequate.

Note: In several cases, I refer to these recipes as *alternatives to insecticides*. They are not necessarily "insecticides" themselves. The government has strict regulations about what you can and cannot call an insecticide for commercial use. Soap, for instance, is very effective at killing some small insects but cannot be *labeled* as an insecticide because it is not registered with the government as one.

"The fact that a pesticide is registered with the government is no guarantee of its safety," according to the National Coalition Against Pesticide Misuse.

The Environmental Protection Agency (EPA) does its best to determine whether a pesticide is safe for public use, and a certain amount of scientific data is required before registration can take place. Unfortunately, the EPA is not always provided with accurate research data. In fact, in 1981, three high-level executives from a contract laboratory—Industrial Bio-Test (IBT) of Northbrook, Illinois—were convicted for providing fraudulent or fabricated pesticide health and safety test data to the EPA.* It has been estimated that at that time IBT performed 30% to 40% of the toxicological studies in the United States. IBT's research supported the registration of at least 325 chemicals for use in a wide range of consumer products: insecticides, herbicides, food additives, chemicals for water treatment, cosmetics, pharmaceuticals, soaps, bleaches, and even coloring for ice cream. After intensive auditing, the vast majority of their studies has been declared by American and Canadian scientists to be invalid.

---

*Schneider, Keith. "Faking It: The Case Against Industrial Bio-Test Laboratories." *The Amicus Journal, National Resources Defense Council Magazine,* spring 1983:14–26.

More recently, in 1994, the owner of another laboratory, Craven Labs in Austin, Texas, has been convicted of falsifying tests conducted for companies seeking registrations with the EPA.*

Does the EPA then consider the registrations for those chemicals to be invalid?† Once a chemical has an EPA number, it's hard to take it away. At that point, unfortunately, chemicals are usually assumed innocent until proven guilty. That means that until you can prove that it is a public health hazard, it may stay in your food, in your water, and in your cleaning products.

Some companies could care less about public health. Keeping that kind of greed and corruption in check can be a difficult and monumental task for a governmental organization. As consumers, we have the responsibility to make sure that the products we buy are adequately proven to be safe. *Purchasing is power.* Use it wisely.

Suffering from an Ant Attack?

There are certain times when ants like to invade our homes: when it's hot and dry and when it's soggy and wet. You don't need to pollute your house with insecticides to keep them out. A simple solution of soap and water will stop them in their tracks. Now you can send those ants to "heaven."

*Hutton, Margaret. "Craven Criminal Case Shows Glitches in Lab Enforcement." *The Daily Environment Report,* Bureau of National Affairs, Inc., Washington, D.C. 1994:1060–2976.

†"Public Health Implications of Alleged Pesticide Data Manipulation by Craven Laboratories, Inc." *For Your Information: Prevention, Pesticides and Toxic Substances* (H75506C) Environmental Protection Agency, Washington, D.C. Sept. 1992.

Amazing Ant Cleaner™

Alternative to Insecticides for Crawling Insects

One August, we had a 100° heat wave in Southern California. It was like a furnace outside, and everyone, including the ants, wanted to stay inside. I had several troops of ants exploring my kitchen and another battalion traversing the door sill. First, I used my Amazing Ant Cleaner™ around the door and along the ant trails on the outside walk. Then I sprayed the ants on my counters. The soap stops them in their tracks and cleans up those "moving pieces of dirt" quite nicely. You can use it to clean up other crawling bugs, too!

Ingredients: Liquid soap or hand-dishwashing detergent and water.

What Else You'll Need: A 16-oz. spray-bottle with an adjustable nozzle.

How to Make: Fill the spray-bottle with water. For this recipe, you can use either liquid soap or detergent. Add 3 tbsp. liquid soap *or* 1 tbsp. liquid detergent. A peppermint- or eucalyptus-scented soap works nicely. The liquid hand-dishwashing detergent at your sink works great, too, but use only 1 tbsp. If you are spraying in environmentally sensitive areas like outdoors, it's kinder to use a liquid soap. Shake to mix.

How to Use: Spray this solution directly on the ants. It works within a few seconds. The soap dries them up. Spray more if needed, then wipe up. This formula is good for many other crawling insects, too.

The five easy steps to an ant-free home are these:

1. Find out what the ants are attracted to and clean it up. Use Amazing Ant Cleaner™ to help clean up the sweet or greasy things. *But don't inhale the soap spray.* Sometimes, the soap sprayed into the air will make you cough or sneeze. Avoid breathing it. Soap spray is good for drying up the ants but not so great for you to breathe.
2. Trace the line of ants to find where they got into the house. Plug up the entrance with petroleum jelly. If the jelly gets

dirty, ants get in. Refresh with a new glob when necessary (or use a caulking gun to seal the hole permanently).

3. Spray the line of ants with soap spray and wipe up. Once you've cleared the house, make sure to squirt every ant that comes in for the next 3 or 4 days.

4. If you plugged up the hole where the ants got in, you can be sure that they will try to find another way in. For this reason, I always spray my ant-infestation prevention formula, Ant Stay Away (the recipe following this one), on the baseboards or window sills near where the ants got in. if they still won't leave you alone, try the other effective prevention techniques: the Honey Pot (see pp. 173–74) or Peppermint Ball (see p. 175) recipes.

5. Keep sweet things in the cupboard or refrigerator. Cleanliness is next to antlessness.

Effectiveness Rating: 90%

Commercial Brand* vs. Amazing Ant Cleaner™ (17.5-oz. ant and roach killer): $3.89 vs. 4¢. 1 tbsp. liquid detergent costs only 4¢. If you use 3 tbsp. liquid soap, this recipe is still a deal at only 24¢. You'll **save** $3.85 each time you refuse to purchase a chemical pesticide.

Note: For hard-surface floors, use vinegar to kill ants. It works slower than soap spray but is easier to clean up and doesn't make floors as slippery as soap does.

---

*Price comparison with Raid.

HOW DO YOU FEEL ABOUT SPRAYING THOSE TOXIC INSECTICIDES IN YOUR KITCHEN OR CHILD'S ROOM?

I bet you're not thrilled when insecticides are sprayed where you and your family can breathe them. Now you have a safe, effective, and even pleasant solution to many of your home insect problems. Most people are amazed that such an alternative exists. I converted all of my neighbors to my ant-control program by giving away spray-bottles of soap and water. They adored me for it.

Amazing Ant Cleaner™ will *not* prevent ants from coming in. Follow my Ant Stay Away and Honey Pot recipes for that. And don't forget that Amazing Ant Cleaner™ works on other bugs and things, too. Try it on any crawling bug or insect. I haven't tried it on them all, but I've used it on silverfish, spiders, pincher bugs, and small roaches. If the liquid soap and water isn't working on your particular insect, try using a liquid hand-dishwashing detergent instead and increase the detergent amount to 2 or more tablespoons. It's also great as an all-purpose cleaner. I use Amazing Ant Cleaner™ for counters, refrigerator, tables, and dishes. I've even used it to squirt my 2-year-old's little hands clean. You certainly can't do that with your ordinary commercial insecticide!

GETTING FLYING INSECTS

I usually get flying insects out of the house by opening a door or window. If it's nighttime, I might turn all the lights out, turn a porch light on, and try to lure the bug out with the light. If you *must* spray something at a flying insect, such as a wasp or bee, please don't use an insecticide. I hate to suggest this, but if you are desperate, you could try using hair spray to immobilize its wings instead.

WHY PAY FOR PESTICIDES WHEN YOU CAN USE PLAIN SOAP AND WATER?

On my last shopping trip, I saw a woman with nothing else in her cart but four beautiful, tall cans of Raid. She paid over $20 for them at the cash register. She had an insect problem and had decided she was going to solve it. It's scary, isn't it? All those ants trooping in to take your food, roaches skittering everywhere, spiders dropping in the night. "Ants!" I can still hear my neighbor screaming. And, now Black Flag comes in all those lovely fresh scents—lavender, pine, even spring fresh. . . . Why not use it as an air freshener?

That thought makes me sick, and rightly so: pesticides can and do make chemically sensitive people sick. I consider chemically sensitive people to be like the coal miners' canary; they are the sensitive indicators of chemicals that I might need to avoid but may not detect myself.

Here are eight reasons why I don't use any insecticides:

1. I can smell them. They make my eyes watery, puffy, and twitchy. I don't like that feeling, and I certainly don't want my toddler to have it.
2. When I use a liquid soap and water spray instead, I save myself over $3 each time I refill the bottle.
3. I'm not afraid of ants and other bugs. I respect them. Insects are an important part of our ecosystem. Ants clean up decomposing, icky messes and turn it into dirt. Spiders eat other insects, keeping insect populations down. I don't want to kill all the bugs in the world; I just want them out of the house.
4. Insecticides don't just stay in the can. The cans get dumped and leak eventually, and the insecticides mix with other chemicals in the landfill. Poisons like this can kill beneficial insects and organisms, disturbing the ability of things in the landfill to decompose organically, and ruin the groundwater. *When we finally get around to cleaning up those landfills, we are going to find out how expensively toxic the products we've been dumping into our garbage really are.*
5. Wherever an insecticide is produced, there may be a dangerously high concentration of it that poses a hazard to local air, ground, and water, particularly if an accident should occur. What about the workers who come into contact with it and their cancer risks? I care

about those people. They could be making soap and water instead.

6. How many cans of insecticide are sold a year? Millions? Where do all those cans go? In the trash. What a toxic mess. Eventually, my taxes are sure to go up from the costs of handling this kind of trash. I can easily refill my spray-bottle with soap and water.

7. How many trucks are on the highway transporting those insecticides? I have a real sense of fear when I drive behind a truck that has those warning signs: Poi-

---

Ant Stay Away

Ant-Infestation Prevention Formula

Use this ant-prevention formula in the areas of your house that are hard to reach and where the ants are getting in. Ants don't like the peppermint scent* and stay away as long as the scent lasts.

Ingredients: Peppermint oil and water.

What Else You'll Need: A 16-oz. spray-bottle.

How to Make: To prevent ants from getting in the house, fill the spray-bottle half full with water. Add 2 tsp. peppermint oil. Shake.

How to Use: Spray the solution where ants come in, on corners, baseboards, window sills, and behind appliances. When hoards of ants were descending upon our kitchen in groups from every which way, this fragrant formula helped to keep them away. I had to *apply it several times over several days* to keep the odor strong.

Effectiveness Rating: 55%

---

*The peppermint scent has not been scientifically proven to repel ants or any other insect; it is simply my personal observation that it does so. A few scientists are testing the insecticidal properties of some essential oils, but we may have to wait many years before we can see the resulting products on the shelves.

son, Flammable, Hazardous Material. The more trucks like that we get off the highway, the safer I will feel.

8. I generally do not support the use of *any* pesticide because no one really knows the long-term effects of exposure to pesticides. Most of the pesticides on the market today have not been adequately tested for long-term effects like cancer and birth defects. Over 50 pesticides have been banned or restricted from use in the United States. Why wait to find out about the next hundred?

The Honey Pot
Ant-Infestation Prevention Formula

"This is for ants, silly, not for bears."

Ants really aren't that bad as long as they stay out of the house. If the last two ant-prevention formulas didn't work, then try this effective diversion technique. Lead your ants to a bowl of sweet nectar, and they'll forget about your house!

Ingredients: Honey and other sweet stuff that ants like, and water. If you have grease-loving ants, then greasy stuff, of course.

What Else You'll Need: A homemade honey pot for the ants. A small paper bowl or cup is fine.

How to Make: Mix ½ cup water with ¼ cup honey and other sweet stuff, such as sugar, corn syrup, maple syrup, fruit juice concentrate, or candy, in a small bowl or cup. Set it outside to distract the ants from invading your kitchen.

What to Do:

1. Make a honey pot for your ants. A small paper bowl or cup will do. If you have pets, you'll need to place it where the ants can get to it but the pets can't. Arranging a mound of rocks around the pot will often do the trick. If you are

inventive, you can make a pretty little pot with holes that the ants can get into but pets can't.

2. Find an ant path outside that you know leads into the house. Sprinkle a trail of sweet stuff on the path and lead them to the honey pot. Once they've found it, they will be delighted with you. Now that you've captured their interest, you can start moving the pot to wherever it is that you don't mind the ants living. Move it gradually, or they will get confused and go back to their food or water source in the house. If the honey pot is crawling with ants and you are afraid to move it, make another fresh honey pot and try to lead them to that one. Dragging a honey pot around with a stick is an acceptable way to move it. Dragging it assures that a lovely sweet trail is left so that the ants know where to find the new location.

3. Refill and freshen the honey pot as needed. Sometimes just adding a bit more water will renew it. Every time you refill the honey pot, try a new sweet treat. Ants are like anybody else and like variety in their diet. Use sweet stuff you might otherwise throw away: half-eaten Popsicles, old Halloween candy, leftover cake icing, and pieces of fruit are all great ant-feeding possibilities. Herding ants like this can be quite a satisfying endeavor. As soon as you start feeding those ants and they start leaving your house alone, you will start to love them. It's the natural way.

Effectiveness Rating: 90%

Here is a letter I wrote one day to my neighbors after a nasty concentrated cloud of pesticides was sprayed right outside my door and my daughter's window without my permission. The pesticide smell lasted for several hours at least, and who knows how long-lasting the chemical residue might be.

Dear Neighbors,

It is the hot and dry season, and ants love to come indoors for food and water. But pesticides are dangerous inside and out.

Peppermint Ball
Ant-Infestation Prevention Formula

Keep those ants dancing with this terrific scented prevention formula.

Ingredients: Cotton balls and peppermint oil.

How to Make: Dip several cotton balls in peppermint oil and rub where you don't want the ants to come in.

How to Use: Ants find their way into your kitchen by following scented ant trails. Use undiluted peppermint oil to confuse their noses. Dip cotton balls into pure essential peppermint oil and wipe along the ants' entrances and paths. The once-organized army of ants will instantly scatter into a confused array. This is the time to eliminate them. Clean up every ant you see; otherwise, they will inevitably find a new way into some delectable treat!

Effectiveness Rating: 70%

"A highly increased risk for leukemia was found for children whose parents used pesticides in their home before giving birth. Home pesticide use resulted in a risk some four times higher than normal for child-hood leukemia. The risk was some six to seven times higher for children of parents who used garden pesticides. The risk was greater with more frequent use."*

Don't use pesticides. I have discovered an alternative that is easy to use: liquid soap and water in a squirt bottle! For the liquid soap, you can use your liquid hand-dishwashing detergent on your kitchen sink. It is safe and works great. But it's not a miracle,

---

*Steinman, David, and Samuel S. Epstein, M.D. *The Safe Shopper's Bible: A Consumer's Guide to Nontoxic Household Products, Cosmetics, and Food.* New York: Macmillan, 1995.

and you do have to keep after the ants. Once you have cleared the house, make sure to squirt and kill every scout ant that will come in for the next 3 or 4 days. And be sure not to leave out any sweet items those ants might enjoy, such as little pools of juice, sponges or rags with juice or food on them, maple syrup, etc.

I'm trying to discourage you from calling [the apartment complex] management and asking them to spray for ants. The spraying is not very effective anyway. When it's hot and dry, ants come in, and when it rains, they are flooded out of their homes and come into yours. You can try to minimize [the likelihood of] ants coming in, but to get rid of the ants completely is sometimes just a matter of waiting out the weather. Put sweet things in jars or in the refrigerator. Don't leave dishes around or garbage inside. If necessary, put it outside on the porch for the night. Ants are a nuisance, but they're not dangerous. Pesticide spraying could be dangerous to your health. Don't ask for it. Because a neighbor had requested it, the pest control man came and, without my permission, sprayed right underneath my 2-year-old's window. The pesticide came into her room in a cloud. He was wearing a mask, but she wasn't. I think this is a crime and a violation of our personal health rights. If you have already called management, please call them up and cancel your ant spraying and try my alternative first. It works on silverfish and other small bugs, too!

Call me if you have any questions or if you want a spray-bottle with a nicely scented eucalyptus or peppermint oil soap in it already. I am selling them for $1.00 apiece just to help everyone out and to keep the neighborhood healthy and ant-free!

Sincerely,
Karen Logan

Boil, Boil, Bubble, and Toil

Ant Nest Eliminator

Sometimes it's appropriate that you end the lives of those poor ants. A nest of stinging red ants in your backyard with a crawling baby in your house is one of those times. Here's a couple of ways to handle it nontoxically.

Ingredients: Boiling water, liquid soap or detergent, and some determination.

What Else You'll Need: A bucket.

How to Make: Add 1 cup liquid soap or ½ cup liquid detergent to a bucket of boiling water.

What to Do:

Strategy #1: Try to get them to relocate the nest. If you are like me and you don't like killing anything, you can try relocating the nest first. Pour a bucket or two of cool water on the nest. You will see those ants with all their little eggs come hurrying out. If you want to herd them away, provide a makeshift highway of lumber or logs for them on which they can escape. When flooded, ants immediately try to go up as high as they can. Climbing a tree temporarily is a typical response. Destroy that old nest with a shovel and cover it up so that they won't want to go back.

Strategy #2: Kill them. If you do have a nest of ants that you must get rid of, this is an extremely effective, inexpensive, and easy way to do it. Make up a couple of buckets of boiling, soapy water. I'd use 1 cup of Dr. Bronner's liquid soap for each bucket. Soap is best because it will biodegrade the quickest. Pour the buckets directly on the nest. You'll never see those ants again.

Effectiveness Rating: 95%

Catering to Cockroaches?

Do cockroaches come to wine and dine in your kitchen at night? Cockroaches are scary and almost invincible. We couldn't survive a nuclear war, but they could. It's a war just to get rid of them. Here's what to do to win:

1. *Stop them from getting in.* Caulk, seal, board up, plug . . . do anything to physically stop those armored race car–like, antisocial bugs from getting in. You can be sure they won't come to the front door to ask if they can move in. Roaches like to sneak into the house along the gaps around pipes and electric wiring. Any crack, hole, or crevice is an invitation to this dark-loving creature to dine. Sealing your apartment or home up seems like an impossible job, and often it is. But if you place your caulking gun under the sink, then when those roaches get you mad, you can pull things away from the walls and start plugging.
2. *Starve them.* Keeping food out of their crusty little claws is often the second most effective thing you can do. It's not *really* possible to starve them. Roaches can live for 3 months without food and 1 month without water. Nevertheless, keeping your kitchen corners clean does help. No more free food handouts for those crusty characters! Don't leave pet food out overnight. Keep food (especially starches like breads and potatoes) in the cupboards, glass jars, other sealed containers, or in the refrigerator. Clean up dishes and spills promptly and thoroughly. It is especially important to get at those bits of food stuck behind the stove, refrigerator, and other difficult-to-move items. I consider it a golden opportunity to deep-clean.
3. *Trap them.* "Look, I caught them!" True hunters are proud of their prizes. Making your own traps not only

will get rid of your uninvited guests but is a surprisingly rewarding experience. If you are not the hunting type, buy an already-made-for-you sticky Roach Motel trap or protected bait trap instead.

Catch 'Em and Cook 'Em
Roach Trap

Here's a version of a coffee-can trap that you can leave out overnight to catch many of those buggy roaches.

Ingredients: Petroleum jelly and roach bait (such as bread, dog food, potato, or fruit).

What Else You'll Need: An empty coffee can or some black masking tape and a larger-size jar.

How to Make: Use a coffee can, or if you use a jar, you will need to cover the outside with black masking tape. Any small- to medium-size container that is dark inside will do. Inside the can or jar lip, smear a generous 2-in. strip of petroleum jelly.

How to Use: Put the jar on its side on the floor, insert bait (bread, dog food, potato, or fruit), and place a cardboard ramp up to the jar lid so that the roach can climb in. The end of the ramp should sit about 1 in. up from the edge of the can so that roaches can get in but not out. Petroleum jelly is too sticky for them to crawl over. Refresh the bait and petroleum jelly as necessary. The trap supposedly works even better once a couple of roaches have fallen in. Just kidding about the "cook 'em."

Effectiveness Rating: 80%

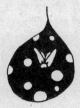

What to Do About Fleas

Fleas are dirty, uncomfortable, and a nuisance. Try these simple alternatives:

1. Vacuum regularly—and keep vacuuming. Bring the vacuum outside and immediately empty the bag every time you vacuum. Otherwise, the eggs stay in the bag and simply hatch in your closet.
2. Don't let your pet go where you can't vacuum or clean. If your pet sleeps on the couch, be sure to use the attachments to vacuum those areas. Train your pet to sleep in one area that you can clean easily and regularly. Hard surfaced floors are the best. Don't forget to wash that bedding.
3. Give your pet a bath. Rumor has it that peppermint- or eucalyptus-oil soap(s) work great in the war against fleas. Dry, flaky skin attracts fleas, so using a mild, conditioning shampoo could certainly help. There are also several natural flea-control shampoos available in most health-food stores.
4. Use a flea comb. As you comb, dip the comb in a bowl of warm, soapy water to kill the fleas and then wipe with a cloth to clean off the dead fleas and eggs.

Here's how washing that dog compares in price to using a flea spray.

Commercial Brand* vs. Wash That Dog (5-oz. flea spray): $7.99 vs. $2.40. Wash that dog with 3 tbsp. liquid soap in 32 oz. of water and it will cost 48¢. Estimate five sprays from a 5-oz. can against five shampoos, and your nontoxic total is $2.40. You'll save $5.59 each time you purchase.

*Price comparison with flea-killer dog spray.

A Mouse in the House

Some mice discovered a bag of bird seed I had stored in my laundry room. This is how I handled it nontoxically:

1. I cleaned up the chewed-on bag of bird seed and put it in a big plastic container, one with a tightly closing top, from which I could easily pour the bird seed.
2. I swept the floor, squirted on a tea tree oil–scented soap, and finished with a peppermint-scented vinegar rinse. The area was clean and smelling fresh. Now, what to do about the mouse? I don't like to kill living things. I also don't like dead ones collecting bacteria and causing odors. Fortunately, I was prepared. I had bought a Smart Mouse Trap from a company called Real Goods (see Resources section, pp. 283–89). This trap catches the mice alive. I got to put it to the test. The instructions said to use a cracker with peanut butter on it for bait. The trap has a little green plastic door with a spring that snaps closed when the mouse tries to eat the cracker. A day later, I checked the trap—dead mouse. He had eaten the cracker and died in his little house from lack of food. I resolved to check the trap sooner next time. From then on, I started catching live mice and setting them loose into the fields in back of where I live. My daughter and I had a lot of fun letting them go and watching them scurry down the path—problem solved.

Are Creepy Crawlers Destroying Your House Plants?

A simple, diluted soap spray is excellent for getting rid of a variety of insects that attack plants. There are special insecticidal soaps on the market especially for this purpose. Safer is a good brand. Although I find it easier and less expensive to simply mix up this recipe myself with a

The Best Bug Spray for Plants

Alternative to House and Garden Bug Sprays

This recipe works great to clean up and control spider mites, aphids, thrips, and other common garden pests. The gardeners I know swear by this simple use of Dr. Bronner's peppermint-scented liquid soap. And this is a great price savings! By making your own spray, you'll save almost $8.00 every time you refuse to purchase another house and garden pesticide.

Ingredients: Dr. Bronner's peppermint-scented liquid soap and water.

What Else You'll Need: A 16-oz. spray bottle.

How to Make: Fill your spray bottle with water (purified when possible). Add 1–2 tsp. Dr. Bronner's peppermint-scented liquid soap. Shake. To prevent sudsing, add the soap *last*.

How to Use: Look for the bugs on the plants and spray the soap directly on them. Those bugs won't live to tell about this soap bath. Most insects are very thin-skinned and cannot tolerate soap; it dries them up. A peppermint-scented soap is even better because the peppermint scent is rumored to repel many insects. Don't forget to check for bugs underneath the leaves and inner stems—spray and wash them wherever you see them.

Effectiveness Rating: 95%

Commercial Brand* vs. the Best Bug Spray for Plants (11-oz. house and garden bug spray): $5.45 vs. 13¢. 2 tsp. liquid soap will cost 13¢. If you use a liquid detergent, 1 tsp. costs less than 2¢. You'll **save** $5.32.

---

*Price comparison with Raid House & Garden Bug Killer.

liquid castile soap that is gentle to my plants. You can use hand-dishwashing liquids as well for this purpose, but detergents are much harsher on your delicate plants. But if your plant doesn't like water sprayed on it, it won't like this solution, either.

Hot Bugs

A Spicy Bug Repellent Alternative to House and Garden Bug Sprays

There are lots of fun homemade formulas for insect repellents that use spicy, repellent ingredients such as garlic, onions, hot peppers, and horseradish—even pulverized bugs! Here is a simple one that uses Tabasco sauce.

Ingredients: Liquid soap, water, and Tabasco sauce.

What Else You'll Need: A 16-oz. spray-bottle.

How to Make: Add 2 tsp. Tabasco sauce to the standard 2 tsp. liquid soap in the Best Bug Spray for Plants. Spray the mixture onto leaves and around the base of the plant. Tabasco sauce repels insects and is stronger and lasts longer than just a peppermint scent. When you use this spray, you've not only gotten rid of the bugs on your plant today, but you've discouraged them from coming tomorrow. That's being nice to you and nice to the environment. Tabasco sauce is a powerful acid and a red-hot bug repellent, but don't use too much or you can burn the leaves!

Effectiveness Rating: 60%

Commercial Brand* vs. Hot Bugs (16-oz. bug repellent): $4.69 vs. 28¢. 2 tsp. liquid soap costs about 8¢; 2 tsp. Tabasco sauce costs about 20¢. You'll **save** $4.41.

*Price comparison with d-Con crawling bug killer.

Kitchen Cleansers

What's Really in Them?

Ingredients in many kitchen cleansers include ammonia, chlorine bleach, dyes, detergents, and trisodium phosphate. They can also contain silica, talc, and oxalic acid.

What Harm Can They Do?

I thought kitchen cleansers were fairly safe. I was surprised to find out that some cities considered cleansers to be hazardous waste. Often, it's the bleach in those cleansers that makes them hazardous. Bleach in any product makes it technically hazardous and a potential problem in the garbage truck and landfill. At home, bleach is hazardous in cleansers because many people unknowingly combine them with other household cleaners containing ammonia, creating toxic chloramine gas. In addition, some heavy-duty cleansers can contain oxalic acid to help them remove rust stains. All this means that kitchen cleansers are not as safe as they seem. Most are harsh and irritating to the skin. Some cleansers will ruin your silver rings, scratch your pearls or opals, discolor your stainless steel, dull your copper, and scratch your Fiberglas. I avoid all these problems by substituting safe, nontoxic baking soda instead.

My friend, Jessica, wanted to clean a spot on her carpet. As many people do when cleaning, she just grabbed whatever cleaning product was around to see if it would get the spot out. She started with ammonia. No luck. The spot was still there. "I'll try some kitchen cleanser," she exclaimed. Dusting the carpet with chlorinated cleanser right on top of the ammonia-soaked spot, she got a cloud of ammonia-chloride gas straight up her nose and screamed. She ended up at the hospital with severe burns on the inside of her nose and throat.

People will try anything to clean up a spot. Please, don't ever mix an ammonia-based cleaner with a cleanser containing bleach. Don't mix an acidic cleanser with chlorine bleach either. *It can produce chlorine gas, which was used in World War I for chemical warfare.* You don't have to go to war just to take out a stain.

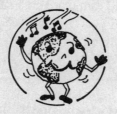

EarthShaker™
Kitchen Cleanser

This is the sweetest and simplest of all my recipes, and the one I use the most.

Ingredients: Baking soda and an essential oil for fragrance.

What Else You'll Need: A plastic flip-top or stainless-steel (powdered sugar) shaker. I reuse a plastic (not cardboard) Kraft Parmesan cheese container. It's a great shaker with a flip-top lid. But be sure to remove the wrapper so that no one mistakes it for cheese!

How to Make: Fill the shaker half full with baking soda. Add 15–20 drops of pure essential lemon or lime oil. Stir. Fill the shaker to the top with more baking soda. Put the lid on the shaker and shake it.

How to Use: Sprinkle EarthShaker™ lightly on counters, sink, or tub, then wipe with damp sponge. Rinse well. Baking soda is a grease cutter, natural deodorizer, and a mild abrasive that will not scratch. Don't shake on too much or you may need a second rinsing. Baking soda is very gentle to the skin, gentle to the environment, and safe to have around the house. Use it on any flat surface that needs to be cleaned and any pot that needs to be scrubbed. It's good for getting scuff marks off the floor, too. *Don't use baking soda on aluminum pots and pans.* If it is left on them for very long, it will turn the aluminum a discolored brown or dark gray.

Effectiveness Rating: 80%

Commercial Brand* vs. EarthShaker™ (14-oz. kitchen cleanser): 57¢ vs. 50¢. 2 cups baking soda costs about 50¢. This is the unscented formula. You'll **save** 7¢ each time you refill the shaker—not much of a savings, but you have a much friendlier product.

---

*Price comparison with Ajax.

Baking soda can clean, neutralize, balance, and deodorize all kinds of oils, soils, and chemicals. You'll love it. A delight at your kitchen sink, this natural mineral is good for 1,001 uses.

Use it for:

- Greasy pots, pans, hands, and dishes
- Getting scuff marks off the floor
- Cleaning and deodorizing your cutting board
- A great scrub for stainless steel
- Softening and dissolving black, burned-on food spots on pots and pans
- Cleaning and deodorizing picnic coolers, lunch boxes, and thermos bottles
- Deodorizing any funny smell in the sink
- A first-aid for bug bites
- A fire extinguisher for oil fires on the stove

Since I started using baking soda at my sink, my sponges always smell delightfully fresh.

Make some lovely baking soda scents. Several boxes of nicely scented baking soda are an absolute cleaning essential in my house. Take a look at my scented baking soda recipes (see pp. 247–52). For kitchen use, my favorite scents for EarthShaker™ are lemon and lime, but I also use lavender, strawberry, apple, and even peppermint. Now, that I've switched from commercial cleansers to scented baking sodas, I could never go back.

A friendly warning: The first time I used baking soda, I was so excited about it that I poured it straight from the box onto everything. It took a lot of work and water to rinse it all off and left an annoying residue. If you use it straight from the box, it's easy to use too much. Just sprinkle lightly. Getting the right kind of shaker helps. Occasionally, I have a bit of leftover residue in a corner, stovetop burner holes, or counter cracks. For these, I squirt on a scented vinegar, and the baking soda dissolves away. A delightfully scented vinegar makes things smell fresh, too.

Getting the right kind of shaker can make a difference in how happy you are with baking soda as a cleanser. I didn't really like baking soda as a cleanser until I got the right kind of shaker. Here are a few options:

1. *Reuse.* I usually don't suggest this, but I make an exception in this one case. The shaker I like the best is a *reused* Kraft Parmesan cheese container (the clear plastic kind with the green top, not the cardboard kind). Make sure to remove the label so you don't have to worry about someone mistaking the baking soda for cheese. Fortunately, it peels off easily. The size is easy to refill and large enough so that you don't have to refill it that often. The bright-yellow top has just the right size holes and an extra flip-top pour side. My assistant, Bonnie, just got an old glass jar with a metal top and poked holes in the top with a nail and ham-

mer. I don't recommend doing this, but I thought it was resourceful and inexpensive.

2. *Get a labeled shaker from me.* You can get a shaker container with the EarthShaker™ recipe right on the label from me at Life on the Planet.

3. *Get an 8-oz. Rubbermaid Servin' Saver with a flip-top lid, found in the plastics aisle of your supermarket.* This shaker has two sides to the flip-top: one for the sprinkle, the other for a real pour. The 8-oz. size is somewhat small for kitchen use. You can switch the top on the 8-oz. shaker to fit the 16-oz. Rubbermaid Servin' Saver drink mixer. I did this, and now I have a larger kitchen shaker that is long lasting and works well.

4. *Use a powdered-sugar shaker.* You can use powdered-sugar shakers to get started with using the baking soda, but the sprinkle is too light and the holes are often too small and get clogged.

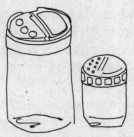

16- or 8-oz. shakers

Because EarthShaker™ is so safe and does not contain any bleach, *it will not remove stains.* If you want to, you can save your old cleanser to use *just* as a stain remover and use the baking soda for all your everyday cleaning. I never use commercial cleansers even for stains—but that's because I know about this absolutely amazing natural stain remover . . .

A Walk in the Park

Stain Remover

For stains on porcelain tubs or stainless-steel sinks, try this naturally acidic and effective formula. It's effortless.

Ingredients: A fresh lemon or lime and baking soda (or salt).

What Else You'll Need: A stain.

What to Do: Wet the stain and pour on the baking soda (or salt). Squeeze on the lemon or lime juice; if you like you can save the rind. Let this solution sit for several hours or overnight. Finish by rubbing with a sponge or the leftover rind. Wash off the stain. This formula usually takes off about 80% or more of the stain on the first try. Repeat the process again, if necessary. If the stain is on the side of a sink or tub, make a sticky, salty lemon paste that won't slide off the stain by adding a little bit of flour. *Salt can scratch, so don't rub too hard.* For more sensitive surfaces and around metal, be sure to use the baking soda for a softer, less abrasive paste.

Effectiveness Rating: 80%

RUST STAINS ON YOUR PORCELAIN TUB OR STAINLESS-STEEL SINK?

Someone left a cast-iron pan sitting in water in our stainless-steel sink. In the morning, there was a beautiful brown rust stain where the pan had been. Of course, my nontoxic EarthShaker™ recipe couldn't take it off, so the stain sat there for a couple of days. On Sunday morning, I decided to get rid of it. I wet the sink, poured salt on the stain, and squeezed a lime over it. It took hours for that rust stain to develop, so I didn't mind that it might take a few hours to get it off. We went out for a walk around the park, played a little tennis, had lunch, and came home. The rust was gone. Aren't nontoxics wonderful? That rust solution cost me about 6 cents and very little effort. By contrast, if I did it the toxic way, I might have tried to use a commercial rust remover like Whink Rust Stain Remover. It contains diluted hydrofluoric acid, which, if it comes into prolonged contact with your skin, can penetrate deeply and if untreated can cause tissue damage until it reaches the bone, where it may start to dissolve that. No one ever uses up all the rust remover in a bottle anyway. It just becomes dangerous, expensive, hazardous waste sitting around in someone's garage. The last Poison Control Center official I talked to about the dangers of products containing hydrofluoric acid knew of a small child who died from ingesting it in his poison control area. The manufacturers of Whink Rust Stain Remover have added a number of child-protective measures to the product in recent years. They point out that Whink can be effectively washed off with water if detected before prolonged and extensive exposure. I'll take the inexpensive, nontoxic lime-and-salt way any day.

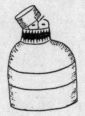

CUTTING BOARDS NEED CLEANING!

Baking soda is great for cleaning your kitchen cutting board, but after cutting raw meat, chicken, or fish on it, you need to think about disinfecting it. Serious disease-carrying bacteria like *Salmonella* can grow in the grooves and crevices of your board. In hot weather, significant bacteria growth can occur in only a couple of hours. Wooden boards are havens for those buggers, but plastic boards can also foster significant bacteria counts.

If you have a wooden board, rub a little salt and hot water into it, wait 5 to 10 minutes or so, and rinse with vinegar. Those nasty bugs can't survive in a solution of salt.* This simple routine eliminates leftover onion, garlic, and other odors as well. Rubbing your board down with half a lemon and some salt is another clever way to clean it. Over time, the salt will dry out your wooden board somewhat, so be sure to condition it occasionally with an overnight soak in vegetable oil. Simply rub the board with the oil, let it sit overnight, and wipe it off in the morning. If your board has a couple of deep knife grooves, it's a good idea to sand those grooves down so that they don't provide dark, moist areas for those little bugs to grow. After sanding, recondition the board again with oil.

If you have a plastic cutting board, the easy solution is to scrub it well with a liquid soap and rinse with hot water after using it.

◆

Laundry Detergents

What's Really in Them?

Ingredients in laundry detergents can include quaternary ammonium compounds, sodium carbonate (or washing soda), sodium alkyl benzene sulfonate, sodium silicate, bleach, enzymes, and sometimes phosphates.

---

*This is not a method scientifically proven to disinfect. I can't guarantee that every last bug will be gone. However, it is common knowledge that a salt solution is powerfully antibacterial.

What Harm Can They Do?

Since having children and doing laundry go together, unless detergents are put on shelves out of children's reach, many children get into them sooner or later. Because they are often high in alkalinity, they can cause burns even if only a little bit is swallowed. Environmentally speaking, detergents are a major component of our wastewater. The more biodegradable and natural the detergent, the better. The choice to use less is best.

The Disappearing Detergent Test

Do you think that when you wash your clothes all that detergent disappears? Well, guess what: it doesn't. Try this enlightening test. Do a wash load as you usually would. Now turn the machine on again for another full cycle, but don't add detergent. Wash again with just plain water. A few minutes later, take a look under the lid. *Suds!* Lots of them. They're proof of the detergent residue in your clothes. That residue is in your clothes right now, making your skin unnecessarily itchy and dry.

The solution? Use less detergent. Detergent manufacturers can overestimate the amount of detergent you need. They figure out an average between the detergent needs of soft water and hard water and put that amount on the label. If you have hard water, you need more. If you have soft water, you need less. When they tell you what to use, they just might be erring on the side of *more* than less. Better to have too much detergent than too little, right? Wrong. This is what happens: in the wash, a detergent loosens the dirt and actually grabs onto it, to lift it up and out of the clothes. The detergent and the dirt get stuck together. If you use too much detergent, you don't always wash it all out. Now, what happens when you don't rinse out all the detergent? You don't rinse out all the dirt! *Your clothes can actually come out dirtier if you use too much detergent.*

Did you think detergent manufacturers were just being helpful by including those handy little measuring cups and caps? It's easy to fill those cups up with just a little more detergent than you really need. *Most washes need only about half as much detergent as the manufacturer suggests.* This may not be true if you live in a hardwater area, but test it out for yourself. Find out—based on *your water* and *your laundry.* If you have detergent residue, you've probably used *too much!*

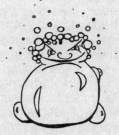

EarthSaver for Your Laundry
Laundry Detergent Helper

I searched and searched for an ecological laundry detergent or soap that worked as well as my favorite detergent. I couldn't find one, but I did come up with this recipe to reduce the amount of detergent I use, and I'm happy about that.

Ingredients: Your favorite laundry detergent and perhaps some baking soda and borax to boost. (You'll find the borax in the laundry section of your store, usually in a green box.)

What Else You'll Need: You'll want to keep a 1/2-cup scooper handy for measuring the baking soda or borax.

How to Use: Use only *half as much* of your favorite laundry detergent as you regularly use. (Please choose a nonphosphate detergent. Check the phosphorus content listed on the label, or simply choose a liquid detergent. All liquids are phosphate-free.) If you need it, instead of adding more detergent, you can add ½ cup baking soda or borax to make your detergent work better. And if you adjust the water level on your washer, make sure to adjust the amount of detergent, baking soda, or borax that you use accordingly. Using only half as much detergent is pretty easy. Using the baking soda and borax is a bit trickier. I've found that I rarely have to add anything to get my laundry clean. Occasionally, I presoak with the baking soda or borax, but that's about it. Remember that *when you reduce the amount of water, you need to reduce the amount of detergent.* Many people don't bother to do this because it's not as easy as turning the dial and sometimes takes a little bit of quick calculating. For small loads, some people add more because it hardly seems like any detergent at all. Other times, they add more just to make sure "it really gets clean." *But remember, using too much detergent actually makes the laundry dirtier!* The warm water and agitation does a lot of the cleaning work. If washers had detergent dispensers that automatically adjusted according to the water level, we would probably use a lot less detergent. If you do need to boost the cleaning power of your detergent, then add ½ cup baking soda or borax along with your regular detergent. When using a liquid detergent, add the baking soda or borax at the same time as your detergent. I keep a box of baking soda and borax right next to my regular laundry detergent.

Effectiveness Rating: 95%

Commercial Brand* vs. EarthSaver (64-oz. laundry detergent): $9.39 vs. $4.69. Tide costs about 22¢ a load. Using half as much of your regular detergent as you normally use will save you from 11¢ to 17¢ a load. Adding the baking soda or borax makes it about a breakeven. There are about 42 loads in a box of detergent. You'll **save** $4.69 each time you buy a box of detergent.

---

*Price comparison with Tide laundry detergent (powder).

Borax for the Laundry

I use borax when my clothes are extra dirty, dingy, oily, or stained. It boosts the cleaning power of detergent, helps to remove soil and stains, deodorizes, and brightens. *Borax is great if you have hard water.* It helps break down the minerals in the water that interfere with the cleaning action of the detergent. Add the borax with your regular detergent at the beginning of the cycle. Borax is particularly effective at removing coffee, tea, and perspiration stains. Presoak with ½ cup of borax and a little laundry detergent.

Baking Soda for the Laundry

I use baking soda when I want to deodorize and soften my clothes. The baking soda helps the detergent work better, softens the water, and leaves your clothes feeling soft and fresh.

- **If you use a liquid laundry detergent:** for a full load, add ½ cup of baking soda at the same time as the liquid. Use less for smaller loads. Don't use too much or you will get an annoying white residue.
- **If you use a powdered detergent:** add ½ cup of baking soda during the rinse cycle. The baking soda will make your clothes softer and cleaner by helping to rinse out the detergent. Make sure to add less for smaller loads.

If you try the EarthSaver recipe for your laundry and the clothes had a powdery residue, use less baking soda and borax. Use ½ cup only for a full-size top-loading machine. If you are doing a medium-size load, use only ¼ cup. For small loads, use just a little shake or two.

How to Make the Change

I find that making any change in my personal lifestyle requires a little bit of effort. Here's how to make this change in your laundry habits easy:

- **Start by using half as much detergent.** Look at the results. If your laundry is like mine, your clothes will be plenty clean with only half as much detergent. If you have extra-dirty laundry, hard water, or your clothes look miserable after reducing the amount of detergent, then go back to the regular amount, but try using less on "light" laundry such as sheets and towels.
- **What about a really dirty load of laundry such as soiled jeans?** Add ½ cup borax as a laundry booster. It works great. Increase the amount of your favorite detergent as you need it. You will be amazed at how for most of your laundry you have been using *twice* as much detergent as you really needed!
- **Washing new clothes for the baby?** Do you worry about those chemical finishes sprayed on new clothes? I used to love that new-clothes smell until I read a report about what's in it: fragranced starches, formaldehyde, insecticides—yuck. Now I presoak new clothes in the washing machine with 1 cup or more of baking soda and then wash them. The baking soda helps to neutralize and remove those nasty and potentially allergenic chemicals. I am especially careful to presoak and prewash my baby's new clothes before she wears them next to her delicate skin.

  CAUTION: Laundry detergents and bleaches are the most commonly reported poison exposures of children under the age of 6. Keep that detergent and bleach on a shelf, please. If you don't have a shelf in your laundry room, now you have a great excuse to go out and get one. And a shelf in the laundry room will make life easier for you.

- **Waste not, want not.** At the end of the life of a bottle of liquid detergent, as much as 1 to 3 oz. of detergent can remain in the cap recesses and at the bottom of the bottle. Don't throw that detergent into the garbage just for it to leak into our groundwater at the landfill. When you're almost finished with the bottle, start the

---

Sweet Pine Tree–Scented Laundry
Alternative Detergent

If you are a purist, you'll want to stop using harsh commercial detergents altogether. Soap flakes are an alternative but hard to get these days. (As of 1991, Ivory Snow isn't soap anymore but detergent.) Try this fantastic formula instead. This environmentally sound alternative detergent was quite a discovery because it's not sold as a detergent but as an all-purpose cleaner. After thoroughly testing it, I was so delighted that I switched from my commercial detergent on the spot.

Ingredients: Dr. Bronner's Sal Suds.

What Else You'll Need: A ¼-cup measuring cup to keep in the laundry room.

How to Use: Use ¼ cup Dr. Bronner's Sal Suds (or 4 tbsp.) for a full load of laundry. Use as you would any other laundry detergent. I've given you the amount I use in my laundry. Add more if you think you need it. Dr. Bronner's Sal Suds is not really a true soap but actually a very refined, specially made biodegradable detergent. The wash comes out incredibly soft and clean, smelling sweetly of pine. It works well in both hard and soft water. Beware: once you try it, you may never go back to commercial detergents again.

Effectiveness Rating: 95%

washer, fill it up with the water from the machine, shake the bottle, and dump the mixture back into the washer. Every little bit counts.

What makes the Sal Suds smell so sweet? It is scented with a high-quality pine-needle oil. Pine oil comes in several quality levels. Oils are extracted from different parts of the tree: needles, trunk, or stump. As you go up the tree, you get a more refined product. Stump oil is crude; pine-needle oil is refined, expensive, and it smells sweeter.

How did Sal Suds clean in comparison to a commercial laundry detergent like Wisk? We tested Sal Suds against Wisk on white towels smeared with spaghetti sauce, chocolate syrup, peanut butter and jelly, maple syrup, mayonnaise, mustard, ketchup, juice, milk, dirt, and Popsicle. We let the towels and the stains sit for 2 days, then we tried to wash them. Unfortunately, many of the stains remained! Both Sal Suds and Wisk left chocolate, ketchup, mustard, dirt, and Popsicle stains, which demonstrates how important it is to pretreat a stain as soon as possible—and before you wash. The Wisk did a better job with the stains, but only by about 15% to 20%—not enough for me to give up the sweet pine scent of Sal Suds. Besides, should we judge a laundry detergent by how powerfully it removes stains? No! Not when I'm about to tell you all my stain-busting tips next. Do your own laundry comparisons if you like. It's fun and easy to do: grab a couple of old white towels and start smearing. I'd be interested in the results.

Penny Watchers

For you penny watchers, here are the approximate costs per load:

- ¹/₂ cup of baking soda (generic): ~12¢ a load
- ¹/₂ cup of Arm & Hammer Baking Soda: ~20¢ a load
- ¹/₂ cup of borax: ~16¢ a load
- Powdered detergent (Tide): ~22¢ a load*
- Liquid detergent (Wisk clear free): ~33¢ a load*
- Dr. Bronner's Sal Suds: ~50¢ a load (I get a great price on the Dr. Bronner's, at Mrs. Gooch's, for about 33¢ a load.)

You'll **save** 11¢–17¢ a load using half as much of your regular detergent.

---

*There are usually 42 loads in a 64-oz. powdered box of detergent and 16 loads in a standard jug of liquid laundry detergent.

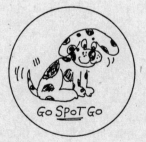

GO SPOT GO

Nontoxic Spot Removers

I used to think that removing spots and stains required nasty, toxic chemicals. Now I know differently. A little detergent, glycerin, and time are all you really need. And, at 52¢ a bottle, the following formula is quite a bargain.

Go Spot Go™

Stain and Spot Remover

When I first tried this formula, I used it on some cotton leggings that my daughter had decorated with red ballpoint pen ink. All of the ink came out beautifully. Then I tried it on some peanut butter and jelly drips smeared and rubbed into her pink ballet leotards and tights. I squirted them with this formula and let them soak for a couple of hours. I came back, and I couldn't believe it: even before washing, the jelly had disappeared! Now I use this spotter on everything—oil stains, spaghetti sauce, chocolate, and ink. It hasn't failed me yet.

Ingredients: Liquid dishwashing detergent *(not soap),* glycerin, and water. I like to use vegetable glycerin, which you can find in some health-food stores. Otherwise, the regular type of glycerin works fine and can be found at many discount pharmacy stores. And be sure to use a *clear,* not colored, liquid dishwashing detergent, like Palmolive or Ivory.

What Else You'll Need: A 16-oz. squirt- or spray-bottle.

How to Make: Mix ¼ cup liquid detergent with ¼ cup glycerin and 1½ cups of water. Pour into a squirt- or spray-bottle; I prefer a squirt-bottle.

How to Use: This "wet spotter" is especially good for ballpoint ink, marker, newsprint, coffee, tea, juice, jams and jellies, barbecue sauce, and mustard. Glycerin has natural stain-removing qualities: it makes that stain so slippery that it just has to rinse out. With the tougher stains, you won't always get all of the stain out, but with a little bit of knuckle-rubbing you'll get at least 50% of it out. You can use Go Spot Go™ on upholstery and carpets as well. Be forewarned: this formula can take a lot of rinsing to get out, so *don't squirt on too much.* Don't use liquid soap for this recipe because it can set sugar and fruit stains. Use a regular liquid hand-dishwashing detergent such as the kind at your kitchen sink. The effectiveness will vary depending on the brand of liquid detergent that you use. So far, I've used Palmolive and Ivory liquids, with great results. I've also used the commercial Spray 'n Wash stain stick for stains and gotten great results. But now that I know how well Go Spot Go™ works, I may never go back.

Effectiveness Rating: 100%

Commercial Brand* vs. Go Spot Go™ (22-oz. spot remover): $2.67 vs. $1.62. Using about ¼ cup liquid detergent will cost you 14¢; ¼ cup glycerin, about $1.48. You'll **save** $1.05 each time you refill the bottle.

---

*Price comparison with Shout.

I bought my glycerin for $2.99 at a local health-food store, but you can also get it at many of the discount pharmacies. Environmentally speaking, it's best to get the natural vegetable-based glycerin. Other glycerins are often made from petroleum—but either kind will work.

What else can glycerin be used for? Why, making bubbles, of course! Go Spot Go™ has doubled as a bubble solution for me many times. It's been a great way to keep my daughter busy while I'm doing the laundry. Here's my official recipe for making bubbles.

More Bubbles, Please . . .

Store-bought bubble solution seems inexpensive but not when you compare it with the homemade kind. I refill my bottles of commercial bubble solution with this formula. I had to include this recipe because it's another way to use your handy glycerin, save you some money, and provide you some fun, too.

Ingredients: Liquid hand-dishwashing detergent and water; glycerin is optional.

What Else You'll Need: An empty jar or bottle to put the bubble solution in.

How to Make: To 1½ cups water, add 3 tbsp. or more of liquid detergent. Add more detergent if your water is hard.

Then add 2 tbsp. glycerin, if you like. The glycerin is supposed to make the bubbles last longer.

How to Use: At our house, we never seem to have enough bubbles: "More bubbles, please, Mommy." One bottle of glycerin and the liquid detergent at your sink is all you'll need for years and years of bubble making. If your brand doesn't work to make bubbles, try another brand. I've used Dove, Ivory, and Palmolive liquids, and they all worked great. The glycerin is supposed to make the bubbles last longer, but I couldn't tell the difference. Perhaps those brands already have enough glycerin in them.

Effectiveness Rating: 100%

Commercial Brand* vs. More Bubbles, Please . . . (64 oz. of bubble solution): $2.99 vs 48¢. 3 tbsp. liquid detergent cost only 12¢. To make 64 oz., you'll need four times the amount in this recipe. Adding the glycerin costs only about 48¢ more. You'll **save** $2.51.

---

*Price comparison with Jack & Jill Bubbles.

Easy Stain-Away
Spot Remover

Vinegar is a mild bleach and works well to help remove some stains. Professionals consider vinegar an essential ingredient in any stain-busting kit. What makes vinegar unique as a spot remover is that it is an acid and tackles alkaline stains that detergents simply won't get out. Having a squirt-bottle of Momma's Earth Mop™ recipe (see pp. 135–36) already under the sink and in the laundry room makes this an easy stain-away.

Ingredients: White distilled vinegar and water.

What Else You'll Need: A 16-oz. squirt-bottle.

How to Make: Fill the bottle half with vinegar and half with water (same recipe as Momma's Earth Mop™).

How to Use: *Vinegar can be helpful in removing the following stains: barbecue sauce, beer, chili, coffee, pet stains, fecal matter, grass, ketchup, orange juice, perfume, perspiration, sour cream, jam or jelly, rust, suntan lotion, tea, urine, and wine.* This recipe works great on grass stains. Detergents actually set a grass stain so that you'll never get them out. If you squirt those green knees and socks with a little vinegar as soon as they happen and let them sit, those grass stains finally come clean! *Don't use vinegar on mustard or blood!* It will set the stain. Get to blood stains right away and use club soda (or *cold* water, not hot) and a mild detergent and a bit of rubbing. A handy bottle of Momma's Earth Mop™ makes it easy to get to stains right away. For many stains, I just grab the bottle from underneath the sink and start squirting, let soak, and wash as usual. One of the keys to stain removal is wetting and rinsing the stain as soon as possible.

Effectiveness Rating: 60%

Do you have a stain that's already set?

If that stain has been around for a while, try this very mild bleaching technique: Squirt Easy Stain-Away on stain, blot dry, rinse with cool water; apply Easy Stain-Away again, dry again; repeat as necessary. Each time you do this, you will bleach the stain slightly. Unlike a chlorine bleach, this method gives you control over the bleaching with little danger of ruining the fabric. Vinegar is safe for most fibers, but it will change the color of some dyes. If you have any doubt, test it on a small area first. But for most permanent stains on whites I still use a dab of chlorine bleach when I have to!

My Tips for Removing Serious Stains

Here's what to do for problem stains:

1. *Get to the stain as quickly as possible.* Just squirt something on it and rinse, even if it's just water. Al-

ways use cool water just to be safe. For laundry stains, I squirt on Go Spot Go™ as soon as possible and let them sit in the laundry room until the next wash. I've also used my handy Momma's Earth Mop™ vinegar recipe in a squirt-bottle to rinse out a stain or carpet spill right away. My club soda glass cleaner works great, too. The longer you let a stain sit without treatment, the harder it is to get out later.

2. *Don't use warm or hot water on sugar stains.* Everybody should know this, but they don't. *Hot water will set a sugar stain;* the heat of the dryer really makes it permanent. For stains from juice, soda, Popsicles, chocolate, candy, coffee or tea with sugar, ketchup, or barbecue sauce: rinse and wash with cool or cold water only.

3. *If the stain didn't come out in the wash the first time, then don't put the clothing in the dryer!* Try a spot remover again, let it soak in, and rewash. Tough stains can sometimes take three or four washings to get out. If you put stained items in the dryer, those stains will be there forever.

4. *For dye, chemical, or colored stains, blot first with paper towels or white rag, rinse, and blot again.* You've probably got a permanent problem. You can try Go Spot Go™, but I don't think the spot will go. Think about getting rid of whatever it was that you spilled that caused such expensive damage. Was it really worth it to have that chemical around?

LM, NO Pee

Or: Look, Mom, No Pee

Is your baby at the age where the pee-pee doesn't always find its way to the toilet? In fact, lots of it gets on clothes, carpeting, couches, and chairs? Try this recipe for a quick, easy deodorizing and clean-up.

Ingredients: White distilled vinegar and an essential oil for fragrance.

What Else You'll Need: Lots of patience and a 16-oz. squirt-bottle.

How to Make: Make up a scented vinegar. Fill a 16-oz. squirt-bottle half with vinegar and half with water (just like my Momma's Earth Mop™ recipe on pp. 135–36).

How to Use: As soon as I can after those accidents, I use tea tree oil– or peppermint-scented vinegar to clean up the spots. In the laundry, I put 1–2 cups scented vinegar in the washer and let the sheets or clothes soak before I wash them. The vinegar actually helps to break down the uric acid in the urine and leaves everything smelling fresh and new. Use this solution to clean up carpet and mattress spots, too. I also use it to quick-clean that potty pot.

Effectiveness Rating: 100%

Metal Polishes

What's Really in Them?

Metal polishes can contain many toxic chemical ingredients. Most contain strong acids such as sulfuric acid, phosphoric acid, oxalic acid, and even dangerous hydrofluoric acid. Other ingredients can include: ammonia, petroleum distillates, nitrobenzene, naphthalene, and ethanol. Less toxic polishes often include detergents, trisodium phosphates, and/or pine oils.

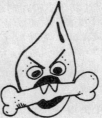

What Harm Can They Do?

Most metal polishes contain acids to dissolve away the tarnish. Those that contain sulfuric or hydrofluoric acid are some of the most dangerous. Even in dilute forms, acids can burn and scar and are especially dangerous to get in your eyes. The hydrofluoric acid found in some rust removers and aluminum polishes is terrifying: if you get it directly on your skin, it can penetrate deeply, robbing your body of calcium and causing tissue damage, and it usually doesn't stop until it reaches the bone! A frightening scenario to say the least.

Other ingredients, such as ammonia hydroxide, petroleum distillates, and ethanol, are powerful skin irritants. If you use them at all, be sure to wear gloves. Many, many polishes are harmful or fatal if swallowed. People report headaches from polishing fumes, but unfortunately, the hazards have undergone little scientific study. Detergents are the least harmful ingredients, but they are also often the least effective. The detergents used in copper polishes can be difficult to wash off completely and cause rapid tarnishing the very next day. Commercial polishes can also damage what you are trying to clean. Dip-type cleaners are notorious for leaving nasty little drip stains on the stainless-steel knife blades of silverware. Others damage finishes.

There are many types of metal polishes, ranging from the fairly safe to extremely dangerous. If you use commercial polishes, please, be kind to your city and the environment, and don't drop metal polishes in the trash. Save any leftover polish for a hazardous waste drop-off.

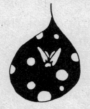

Environmentally speaking, cleaning any metal is somewhat polluting to our water. It's best to ask yourself, "Does it really need to be cleaned?" If you are an environmentally enlightened, lazy type of cleaner like I am, the answer is usually no. Nevertheless, occasionally a few pieces of metal do seem to need polishing, so I've included these quick and easy recipes just for those times. But first, here are my tips for cleaning metal nontoxically:

1. *Natural acids, such as lemon juice or vinegar, combined with salt make great metal cleaners.* Most of my recipes involve a natural acid and a salt to clean the metal: lime and salt for copper; vinegar, flour, and salt for brass. Most any acid will help to clean a metal; you simply need to choose a safe and mild one.
2. *Give these natural metal polishes* time *to work.* Tarnish and metal stains take days—even weeks—to develop. Why should we expect them to disappear in a few seconds? Some of these naturally mild solutions may take a couple of hours or even overnight to work, but it's worth it to keep your family and your environment safe. Patience is, after all, a virtue.
3. *Oil helps keep tarnish and rust away.* Rubbing a tiny bit of oil (any olive or vegetable oil will do) on your

freshly cleaned copper, brass, or silver will help to prevent it from tarnishing again. I usually put a couple of drops of olive oil on a soft, smooth cotton cloth and then rub the metal item with it. It's not a full-proof antitarnisher, but it does seem to help.

I have a few cast-iron cooking pots and pans that I inherited from my grandmother. They're great pots and pans to cook in, but it took me a little while to learn how to clean them. Cast-iron pots, like woks, get better the more you cook in them. These kinds of pots love that dark, built-up layer of stuck-on food that becomes carbon. The black helps the food to cook more evenly, protects the pan, and keeps the food from sticking. The first time I cleaned my cast-iron pots and pans, I let them soak in liquid detergent and let them sit on the rack to dry. Rust! My mother told me later that you don't need to clean them with soap but you do need to condition them with oil and dry them as soon as they are washed. I conditioned and oiled away, and now I hardly ever see a bit of rust. Oil resists water, of course, and it's the water that makes them rust.

Cleaning Brass and Copper

Copper Margarita
Brass and Copper Cleaner

This is my favorite Friday-night "how to entertain the guests with my nontoxic cleaners" recipe. I like to demonstrate on my copper-bottom pots. Try it yourself. You will oohh and aaahh like my guests always do.

Ingredients: One lime or lemon and some ordinary table salt.

How to Use: Cut a lemon or lime in half. Sprinkle a little salt on whatever needs polishing and start rubbing—immediately, you get super results. That's right—the tarnish comes off with just a little lime juice and salt. I prefer to use limes rather than lemons because they don't have any seeds, are easier to rub with, and are a little more effective.

Effectiveness Rating: 90%

Commercial Brand* vs. Copper Margarita (5 oz. of brass and copper cleaner): $3.09 vs. 96¢. Half a lime costs approximately 5¢; 1 tbsp. salt costs less than 1¢. That's 6¢ for one application, and 96¢ for a total of eight applications. Compared with the approximately eight applications you'll get from a 5-oz. jar of Twinkle, you'll **save** $2.13.

---

*Price comparison with Twinkle brass and copper cleaner.

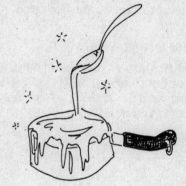

Miracle Metal Goop™
Brass and Copper Polish

Kids love to goop this formula onto your pots, pans, and brass pieces. They will be tempted to eat it, but they won't because it tastes so bad. This is a great recipe for curvy bronze candlesticks and intricate statues.

Ingredients: Flour, white distilled vinegar, and salt.

What Else You'll Need: A large plastic or glass mixing bowl and spoon (don't use a metal pot).

How to Make: Mix ²/₃ cup white distilled vinegar with ²/₃ cup flour. Stir the mixture until smooth. Add ¹/₂ cup salt and stir until mixed in. This formula doesn't keep well, so make a fresh batch each time you need it.

How to Use: Spoon this mixture onto your brass candlesticks, copper pots, and any tarnished brass or copper item. If the goop drips too much, add 1 tbsp. more flour to the mixture. You want to get a nice, sticky, smooth layer to stay on the metal. Miracle Metal Goop™ starts working right away, but you get the best results if you leave it on for 1 or 2 hours or even overnight. You'll know it's really working when the goop starts to turn green. *Green goop is toxic, so don't let the kids get into it.* My rule is that it's okay for the kids to put it on the copper, but I get to take it off. Rinse the copper off well and wipe clean. I finish polishing with a soft cloth and a dab of olive oil. The oil helps to prevent further tarnishing and gives your piece a soft shine.

Effectiveness Rating: 90%–100%

Commercial Brand* vs. Miracle Metal Goop™ (8 oz. of brass and copper cleaner): $3.04 vs. 39¢. 1 cup flour costs 8¢; 1 cup vinegar, 16¢; and ³/₄ cup salt, only 15¢. You'll **save** $2.65 each time you refill the jar.

*Price comparison with Brasso.

If you make Miracle Metal Goop™ ahead of time, make sure that the lid is screwed on tightly when you're finished. Otherwise, your miracle will harden in the jar. I suggest that you make it only as needed. If you do want to keep this paste around awhile, you can cut up a small sponge, soak it in water, and stick it in the jar. The sponge will keep that paste nice and moist for at least a couple of months. Remoisten the sponge as necessary. This is a vigorous-smelling paste, so don't stick your nose straight into the jar or bowl to check it out. A whiff will scrunch your face up.

You may still have black spots on your copper-bottom pots even after using Miracle Metal Goop™. Black, cooked-on spots on copper-bottom cookware are hard to remove. The popular commercial copper polish, Twinkle, won't remove them, either. Try using a bronze wool pad—bronze wool is softer than steel wool—but be careful to work the spots off gently to minimize the scratches. Then, massage those bottoms! I always think of the Coppertone baby's bottom when I do this. Less toxic metal polishes tend to allow tarnish to form again quickly. A loving oil massage for those pot bottoms seems to help a little. Use your handy olive oil and put a little love in it. Better yet, give the environment a real lift and massage somebody you love instead.

What about tarnish on copper and brass plating? Use plain dishwashing detergent or a very mild solution of warm vinegar and a dash of salt. All metal polishes remove some metal while cleaning off the tarnish, so if your piece is a family heirloom, be careful to use a milder solution and work up to the stronger formulas until you find which one is best for that piece.

Brass is often coated with a lacquer to prevent tarnishing. If the lacquer has chipped off and the metal has tarnished below, then the only way to effectively clean the entire piece is to first remove the lacquer. I'd use a little bronze or steel wool before I'd use a toxic chemical lacquer remover. Beware: if you do use steel wool, many items have a thin coat of brass plating and you will end up simply rubbing the brass away. Consider living with the tarnish or replacing the item.

Salty Juice Bath
Brass and Copper Dip

Salty Juice Bath is a handy, effortless brass and copper dip-type cleaner. It's more expensive than commercial dips, but if used occasionally, it's only 7¢ more a dip and saves you the effort of polishing. Also, I found this dip to be quite a bit more effective than commercial ones.

Ingredients: Lemon juice (reconstituted) and salt.

What Else You'll Need: A big pot (to use as a container to hold the dip).

How to Make: Mix ½–1 cup lemon juice (use bottled, reconstituted lemon juice) and 2 tbsp. salt in the bottom of a pan. Fresh lemon juice works best, but really . . . if I took the time to squeeze the lemon juice, I'd use it for fresh lemonade instead.

How to Use: Use this recipe for any brass or copper item you want dipped to a shiny clean. Here's how I clean my copper-bottom pots: I run 2 in. of water in a big spaghetti pot. Then I add 1 cup lemon juice and 2 tbsp. salt. I put the tarnished bottom of the pot I want cleaned into the salty lemon water. Next, I set a glass full of water in the center of the tarnished pot to keep it submerged. The results? Beautiful, shiny bottoms. Finish up by rubbing a little olive oil to prevent future tarnish and give them a nice sheen.

Effectiveness Rating: 80%

Commercial Brand* vs. Salty Juice Bath (~5 oz. of brass and copper cleaner): 39¢ vs. 46¢. One application: ½ cup salt costs 6¢; 1 cup lemon juice costs 40¢. Based on an estimated eight applications in a 5-oz. jar of Twinkle, this cleaner will **cost** you an extra 7¢ each time you use it.

---

*Price comparison with Twinkle.

Now that I've shown you all these very nice ways to clean your copper-bottom pots, I'm going to tell you about the least toxic way: don't clean them at all! It's nice to have shiny copper-bottom pots, but the truly "environmental" thing to do is to not clean the bottoms of your pots and pans at all. The leftover water with the little bits of metal in it is truly polluting. If you hang your pots up for show, you might consider putting the copper-bottomed ones in the cupboard. It's a lot of work keeping those bottoms shiny. Besides, your pots will cook better and more evenly and last longer when they have a nice black bottom. Give it up; the rest of the house needs cleaning.

Cleaning Silver

Tarnish-Away

Silver Polish

Tarnish-Away is a quick and easy way to polish up your good silver at the last minute before the guests arrive. This amazing formula will miraculously magnetize your tarnish away. No more rubbing and scrubbing with toxic polishes; no more dry hands exposed to toxins.

Ingredients: Aluminum foil, salt, and baking soda.

What Else You'll Need: You'll need a container that will hold your silver pieces. Glass or plastic works best. If you have large silver items, you can use your sink. If you use the sink, make sure it is tightly plugged. For small items, a glass or plastic bowl is fine.

How to Make: Put 1 sheet of aluminum foil, 1 tbsp. salt, and 1 tbsp. baking soda into a bowl or large container. Fill the container with warm water. Place the silver into the container. Wait 1 hour, then wipe off silver with a soft cloth.

What to Do: I've used this formula with beautiful, effortless results on my good silver, as well as on several hard-to-polish silver items, such as ice buckets and candlesticks. Make sure to use only glass or plastic bowls to do this. If you use a metal pot or bowl, some of the tarnish can adhere to it. *This formula starts working within a few minutes.* The tarnish comes right off the silver and onto the aluminum, most of it within 1 hour. Rinse and wipe dry with a clean cloth. If a lot of tarnish is being removed, it will smell slightly of rotten eggs. If you do smell rotten eggs, make sure to ventilate the room and turn on your kitchen fan: that odor is hydrogen sulfide gas—toxic if you breath it in a concentrated form. This is why I suggest the slow, leave-it-to-soak method rather than the traditional boil-it-quick method, which releases the gas in a more concentrated fashion. Don't worry; a little bit of this gas is about as toxic as visiting a natural hot spring—but I wouldn't stand over the sink and take a whiff of it, either. If the foil gets dark, replace it with new foil.

Effectiveness Rating: 80%–90%

Commercial Brand* vs. Tarnish-Away (8 oz. of silver polish): $4.07 vs. 30¢ A sheet of aluminum foil costs 3¢; 1 tbsp. baking soda, 2¢; and 1 tbsp. salt, less than 1¢, for a total of 6¢ per application (based on approximately five applications). You'll **save** $3.82 each time you clean.

*Price comparison with Wright's silver cream.

Polishing always takes a bit of the metal away. Tarnish-Away is no exception. Even though it makes silver polishing easy, I wouldn't use this formula regularly or you may damage your silver. It's best to keep your heirloom silver pieces tarnish-free in their tarnish-resistant little cloth bags. If you don't have the bags already, consider buying them. It's your best investment for keeping that silver lovely. If your silver knives have stainless-steel blades, use Tarnish-Away *only on the silver handles*. Put just the handles—not the blades—in the solution.

The Toothpaste Touch

Metal Spot Remover

This isn't a very effective recipe, but it's a handy and appealing one. Toothpaste is a fairly well known home remedy for polishing metals. If you have a choice, use the brightening, whitening kind—I think it works best.

Ingredients: Toothpaste.

What Else You'll Need: A soft cloth.

How to Use: You can take care of those last few dark spots left on your brass, copper, or silver by using a little dab of toothpaste and a brush. Rub it in with your fingers and brush. It's great for the darkened crevices. The toothpaste will help to lighten the dark spots but will rarely take them completely off. Add a couple of drops of olive oil to the paste to increase its effectiveness. Although the toothpaste rates at a low 35% effectiveness at getting those last few dark spots out, it's handy to know that in a pinch, you can use it as a cleaner. Or try a little Tabasco sauce on those spots and let the pieces sit, then brush them. If the spots don't come out, don't dismay. Life isn't always perfect, and neither will your silver be. Delight in the imperfection of life and a life without toxic chemicals.

Effectiveness Rating: 35%

"Har, Har" Jewelry Jar

Silver Jewelry Cleaner

Cleaning jewelry is tricky. Glues dissolve. Stones do get scratched. Gold is soft. Pearls and opals are easily dulled by abrasives. To be safe, clean only silver jewelry with this recipe. For other jewelry, try a little toothpaste and an old toothbrush—or even just a little liquid soap or detergent and water—to clean your gold and diamond rings.

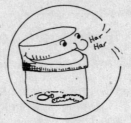

Ingredients: Aluminum foil, warm water, salt, and baking soda.

What Else You'll Need: A glass jar or bowl.

How to Make: In a glass jar, mix 1 tsp. salt with 1 tsp. baking soda. Fill the jar half full with postage stamp–size pieces of aluminum foil. Add warm water. Drop your jewelry in for 15 minutes to 1 hour. Then spoon it out and polish it with a soft cloth. Refresh the ingredients when the aluminum foil starts to turn dark.

How to Use: Use this solution to clean up your silver jewelry. I keep some ready made in a jar under the bathroom sink. *Kids love Har, Har Jewelry Jar as a silver-polishing magic science trick.* They can use it to polish their quarters and dimes. You can use it to make their allowances shiny and special.

Effectiveness Rating: 90%

Cleaning Stainless Steel

Stainless Steel Cleaner par Excellence

I use this recipe regularly on my teapot (that gets greasy on the stove) and my stainless-steel sink (which needs no explanation). Really the EarthShaker™ recipe in disguise, this recipe is yet another reminder that baking soda is great for cleaning any stainless-steel surface.

Ingredients: Baking soda.

What Else You'll Need: The soft side of your sponge.

How to Use: Baking soda is an excellent stainless steel cleaner. Don't use a green-backed sponge, because it may scratch. Eventually all the metal in my house gets scratched one way or another or by someone or another, so I'm not particular. If you are bothered by a white baking soda residue, use a scented vinegar rinse after you've finished scrubbing and you'll never see that white dust again.

Effectiveness Rating: 95%

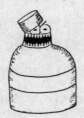

Rust Removers

This story was told to me by Sarah from the Household Hazardous Waste Project in Springfield, Missouri, an excellent consumer-oriented environmental organization. Sarah gives seminars on the hazards of household products. During the seminar's section on rust removers, one of the participants had this true-life tale to tell.

One day, the woman was innocently cleaning the rust off something metal with Whink, a store-bought rust remover containing hydrofluoric acid. She thought she had protected herself by wearing the ordinary yellow latex gloves. Undetected, the rust remover leaked through a small hole in a glove and got on her skin. To her surprise, hours later, her finger started to swell and hurt terribly. She rushed to the emergency room. The hydrofluoric acid in the rust remover didn't stop penetrating until it hit the bone, where it ate away the bone until it was neutralized. Now, she has permanent nerve damage.

Don't trust latex gloves to protect you from dangerous cleaners. They may not be sufficient to protect you, and the gloves could have holes in them that you don't know about. More importantly, I strongly suggest to never, ever use any product that has hydrofluoric acid listed as an ingredient. Hydrofluoric acid is extremely dangerous. On prolonged contact with the skin, the acid can penetrate your skin and muscle until severe tissue damage has occurred. If it has been spilled on a large area such as an

A Walk in the Park

Rust Remover

You've seen this recipe before in the Kitchen Cleansers section (see p. 189) as a general stain remover. Here you see it in its most powerful form as a rust remover. Commercial rust removers can contain dangerous phosphoric or hydrofluoric acids. Now you have an effective, safe alternative.

Ingredients: A lemon or lime and salt, plus a little flour, if necessary.

What to Do: Wet the stain and pour on the salt. Squeeze on the lemon or lime juice. Save the leftover rind. If the stain is on the side of a sink or tub, mix up a salty lemon paste. Add a little flour to make it stickier. Let this solution sit for several hours or overnight. Rub the spot with the leftover rind, then wash it off. This usually takes off about 80% or more of the stain on the first try. Repeat again if necessary. This is also an effective treatment for rust stains on metal surfaces.

Effectiveness Rating: 80%

Commercial Brand* vs. A Walk in the Park (8-oz. rust remover): $2.99 vs. 60¢. A half of a lemon or lime will cost you about 5¢; the salt, less than 1¢. Based on 10 applications per bottle, you'll **save** $2.39.

*Price comparison with Whink.

arm or leg and left untreated for a prolonged period, you could be in serious trouble and could end up in the intensive care unit with a condition called hypocalcemia. Hydrofluoric acid is a poison, and children have died from ingesting it.

Pumice Power

This is another powerful, nontoxic rust remover. You'll see this suggestion in several places: oven cleaning, toilet bowl cleaning, and tub and tile cleaning. The pumice stone is a great cleaning tool for the tough stuff that most people think only chemicals will get out. It's excellent for taking graffiti off, too. It takes a bit of getting used to, but it's really remarkable!

Ingredients: A pumice stone. Get one from your local hardware store or from a cleaning catalog (see Resources section, pp. 283–89).

How to Use: Wet the stone thoroughly and rub. Use it to remove rust stains from any ceramic or porcelain surface like the tub or sink. Don't worry about scratching. The pumice stone is not harder than your porcelain. As long as you keep it wet, it won't scratch. But, please, don't use on metal, Fiberglas, or aluminum surfaces.

Effectiveness Rating: 100%

Oven Cleaners

What's Really in Them?

Oven cleaners can contain sodium hydroxide, potassium hydroxide, and/or ammonia. Other ingredients include methylene chloride, butyl cellosolve, chlorine, and detergents. Most are hazardous to use and dispose of.

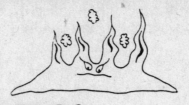

What Harm Can They Do?

The most common and dangerous ingredient in oven cleaners is sodium hydroxide or caustic soda, commonly known as lye. Sodium hydroxide is extremely corrosive and toxic. Even when very diluted, it is hazardous to the eyes, nose, and skin and can cause burning and scarring. Aerosol oven cleaners are particularly hazardous since the chemical vapor is more likely to get into your eyes and lungs. Please, don't dump unused oven cleaner down the drain or into the garbage. Bring it to your local hazardous waste center. (I hope you have one!) Here's what Consumer Reports Books had to say about oven cleaners: "A little dirt in the oven never hurt anybody; a little oven cleaner might."*

There is no doubt that many oven cleaners are dangerous to use—so dangerous that consumer safety organizations suggest that while cleaning an oven you should wear safety goggles to protect your eyes, an apron for your clothes, and protective gloves for your hands. Put layers of newspaper on the floor and avoid breathing the fumes as much as possible.

Why? *The sodium hydroxide present in a typical aerosol oven cleaner will show damage to a healthy lung within 15*

---

*Florman, Monte, and Marjorie Florman. *How to Clean Practically Anything.* p. 71. New York: Consumer Reports Books (a division of Consumers Union), 1993.

Never Clean an Oven Again
Oven Cleaner

There are a couple of great alternatives for cleaning your oven, the most effective of which is prevention. *Try this solution—it's wonderful. I've used it for years.*

What You'll Need: An aluminum oven liner. You can usually find liners in the baking supplies section of your grocery store. If you can't get an aluminum oven liner, you can use a cookie sheet, or in a pinch, aluminum foil.

How to Use: Heaven is never cleaning an oven again. Impossible? Ever heard of an oven liner? It's a thin aluminum cookie sheet–like tray that you put in the bottom of your oven to catch those drips that later become the baked-on nasties. Oven liners are an inexpensive, quick, and easy solution to oven problems. Also, oven liners are pure aluminum, so you can recycle them when you're done. You can also use an old cookie sheet or aluminum foil to protect the bottom of your oven, but cookie sheets warp and foil doesn't always stay where you want it to, so it's better to get an oven liner if you can. But if you've got a gas barbecue grill outside, you can line the bottom of that with a couple of sheets of aluminum foil, which works great. Make sure to poke some holes in the foil so the air vents can work. Now you're ready to Never Clean an Oven Again. **Note:** If you use an old cookie sheet as an oven liner and it gets crusted and icky, soak it overnight in the sink with a paste of baking soda and water. Add a little dishwashing detergent if you like. In the morning, you can scrape and scrub the grime off. Cookie sheets are great to use in a pinch, but it's better to use an oven liner. Cookie sheets are too thick and can interfere with the even heating of your oven.

Effectiveness Rating: 95%

Commercial Brand* vs. Never Clean an Oven Again (16-oz. oven cleaner): $3.52 vs. 75¢. A store-bought oven liner costs only 75¢. The oven liner will probably last longer than the life of the can of oven cleaner. You'll **save** $2.77.

---

*Price comparison of Easy-Off fume free with Handi-foil oven liner.

minutes of use.* That means if you are cleaning with a toxic oven cleaner, don't keep your head in the oven! But, of course, I suggest that you don't clean it at all (see my Never Clean an Oven Again recipe).

My next-door neighbor had just finished moving in, and she turned the oven on for the first time. Within a few minutes, her entire apartment reeked of a horrible chemical smell. I heard her yelling for help. "What happened?" she cried. The people who cleaned the oven last had incorrectly sprayed oven cleaner on the heating elements. Not only does that ruin the oven, but it can release fumes the next time you turn the oven on. I told her to open the windows and doors and get out of the apartment until the cleaner had burned off.

Sleep It Off™
Oven Cleaner

Aerosol oven cleaners can do more than damage your lungs. They can also damage your clothes, floors, counters, and oven. Sprays are easy to misdirect and get on things they shouldn't, such as heating elements, metal trim, plastics, and linoleum. You don't have to use damaging chemicals to clean your oven. With a little patience, you can sleep your oven troubles away.

Ingredients: Salt, baking soda, and water.

What Else You'll Need: A shaker, a mixing bowl, a measuring cup, and a spray-bottle of diluted liquid soap and water.

---

*Harte, Holdren, and Shirley Schneider. "Sodium Hydroxide." In Toxics A to Z. Berkeley: University of California Press, 1991:399.

How to Make: Mix ¼ cup salt with ¾ cup baking soda. Fill the shaker. Use a measuring cup with a pour spout or funnel to make the filling process neater. To make the paste version: add ¼ cup water, mix, and use directly from the bowl.

How to Use:

1. Before doing anything, plug up any holes in the bottom of the oven with foil. This prevents the cleaner from leaking into the broiler area. Spray the oven with water or a diluted soap-and-water spray. Now, shake the salt–and–baking soda mixture on. Spray the oven again with water until the mixture is slightly damp and pasty. For the side walls, make a thick paste in a bowl by adding ¼ cup water to the ¼ cup salt and ¾ cup baking soda. Smear paste on the oven walls with a sponge. Salt can corrode metal, so try not to get it on any metal parts.

2. Now you can go to sleep. Sleep It Off™ works overnight at dissolving those black, baked-on spots. In the morning, get your serious oven-cleaner tools ready: a flat spatula-type scraper (putty knife), green-backed sponges, some fine steel wool (grade 0000), paper towels, sponge or rag for rinsing and drying, spray-bottle of soap and water, and a squirt-bottle of scented vinegar. With the putty knife, scrape off all the goop and pile it onto the paper towels. Use the green-backed sponges or the very fine steel wool next to work off any tenacious spots. Be gentle; you don't want to rub off the enamel! Wipe down the oven with your soap-and-water spray. You may need to do a second rinsing.

3. Finish with a total oven squirt of scented vinegar to dissolve any baking-soda residue. Dry the oven. *Remember to take those aluminum-foil plugs out of the holes in the bottom of the oven.* From now on, use an oven liner so you'll never have to clean an oven again!

Effectiveness Rating: 75%

Commercial Brand* vs. Sleep It Off™ (16-oz. oven cleaner): $3.49 vs. $1.05. Per application, this recipe will cost you ½ cup salt at 6¢ and ½ cup baking soda at 15¢ (compared with approximately five applications in a 16-oz. can). You'll **save** $2.44.

---

*Price comparison with Easy-Off original.

What About Years of Baked-On Stuff?

If you have an ugly, messy oven and you need to clean it quickly, then use *the magical pumice stone* to get rid of those ancient drips. If you don't have a pumice stone, try using a very fine steel wool (grade 0000) pad. I got my pumice stone from one of the cleaning supplies catalogs I have listed in the back of this book (see Resources, pp. 283–89). Always, always *wet* your pumice stone before using. Rubbing the spots with the pumice will make a horrible grating sound, but don't worry. If you keep the stone wet, I guarantee you that it won't hurt your enameled oven. Don't use it on metal parts, though. *You will need to add a little nontoxic* patience *to this recipe to counteract the months and even* years *of oven-cleaning neglect.* Keep working; you will eventually get it off. Tired of scrubbing? Take a break and soak those spots with my Sleep It Off™ paste for at least 30 minutes. Three soaks, a little more rubbing, and it's sure to come off.

You can use Sleep It Off™ for your oven racks, too. Smear on the baking-soda paste. Add a couple of squirts of hand-dishwashing detergent, if you like. Detergents are great for grease. Let the racks soak in the sink or put them in a plastic garbage bag out of the way. The longer they soak, the better. Scrub them with steel wool or a green-backed sponge, rinse with soap and water, give them a final rinse of vinegar, and you're done.

If not rinsed completely, Sleep It Off™ leaves a white residue after it dries. In an oven, it can be hard to rinse off the baking soda completely, but you won't see the residue until it dries. *A quick squirt of scented vinegar will dissolve that white residue,* freshly scent your oven, and help to prevent grease from sticking next time.

If the baking soda clogs your oven's burner holes, squirt a little vinegar on them and that baking soda will dissolve away. If the holes are clogged with soap or other cleanser, then carefully use a paper clip to open them up again.

The Oven-Cleaning Power Tools

Tools are important. If you are a professional or die-hard oven cleaner, you will love this list.

1. *The great glob remover—the putty knife.* Putty knives are available at most hardware stores and through some cleaning-supply catalogs. Use them to scoop and scrape.
2. *Paper towels.* Scooping up yuckies is what I call "the proper use of a paper towel." Grease and blackened food can ruin a cleaning rag. Cleaning an oven is a great use for paper towels; using them to wipe a little water off your hands is a waste.
3. *The pumice stone.* At only about $1 apiece and lasting for 15 to 20 uses, pumice stones are your best friend for tenacious oven spots. They're useful for toilet bowl stains, too.
4. *The razor blade set.* Razor blades can be dangerous. Nevertheless, if used properly, they are effective and nontoxic. They're great for scraping globs off glass oven doors and dried paint off windows. I've never had to use one for cleaning an oven, but some professional cleaners I know swear by them. Please, use them carefully and cautiously.

Oven cleaners are dangerous to use, dangerous to have in the house, and dangerous to dispose of. Why pay money to bring hazards into your life? Now, you can leave them on the shelf. If you have to clean an oven that you think has oven cleaner residue in it, use gloves and first wash it thoroughly with soap and water—*then* start your nontoxic cleaning.

Oven-Cleaning Tips: An Ounce of Prevention Is Worth a Pound of Cure

You won't have to spend much time cleaning your oven if you catch spills early:

- *Afraid to look in the oven to see what has spilled?* Don't be. We all routinely wipe down our kitchen counters. Why not the oven? If I've used the oven, then after dinner, I take care of any fresh oven spills quickly with a sprinkle of Sleep It Off™ or just plain baking soda and a squirt of soapy water. Then I let those spills soak and the oven cool while I wash the dishes. After I've loaded the dishes, I finish by getting that grubby stuff off the oven with a nylon mesh scrubber. It always comes right up.
- *For the yummy lasagna that you're sure will boil over, remember to put your oven liner in.* The spills will go onto the liner, and there's nothing for you to clean up afterward.
- *If you do a lot of messy baking, keep a putty knife near the oven and scrape up spills inside as soon as the oven cools.* If you don't have a putty knife, you can use a metal spatula instead. Be careful not to push too hard or you'll bend the handle.
- *Are there grease puddles?* If they're still warm, ordinary table salt will soak them right up. Sprinkle it on, let the salt sit, then scoop up the grease and finish with a soapy water rinse.

What About the "Fume-Free" Oven Cleaners, Pump-Spray Types, Pads, and Brush-On Jelly Kinds?

Pump sprays are easy to inhale and can be difficult to control. "Fume-free" cleaners come packaged in environmentally unfriendly aerosol cans. Pads containing toxics are expensive and wasteful. Jellies spatter and are time consuming to apply. If you switch to using an oven liner and a little Sleep It Off™, you'll save money and never have to worry about handling toxics again. In fact, you'll save over $10 if you switch from an expensive oven-cleaning pad to a disposable aluminum oven liner. Here's the price comparison:

Commercial Brand* vs. Never Clean an Oven Again (pad oven cleaners): $2.94 vs. 75¢. A store-bought oven liner costs only 75¢. The oven liner will probably last for the equivalent of at least 10 cleanings with pads, compared with only one application per pad package. You'll **save** $2.19 every time you clean the oven; you'll **save** $21.90 over the approximate life span of the oven liner.

*Price comparison of S.O.S Oven Pad with Handi-foil oven liner.

Cleaning Barbecue Grills

Please, take it easy and don't clean the grill at all! That crusty old black carbon on your grill actually helps it cook better and is cherished by barbecue masters. Don't worry about bacteria; the heat of the barbecue sterilizes any leftover food. If the carbon crusts are sticking to your chicken, making it more than Kentucky fried, then take a wire brush to the racks, and then call it a sunny Sunday afternoon.

◆

Toilet Bowl Cleaners

What's Really in Them?

Most toilet bowl cleaners use a strong acid, such as hydrochloric acid or sulfuric acid, to clean. SnoBol (liquid) toilet bowl cleaner contains 15% hydrochloric acid; Lysol brand (liquid) contains 8.5%. Other toilet bowl cleaners, such as Vanish (powder) and Sani-Flush (powder), contain sodium bisulfate. When a powdered toilet bowl cleaner containing sodium bisulfate mixes with water, then sulfuric acid is produced. Other ingredients can include muriatic or oxalic acid, phenols, ammonia, PDCBs, naphthalenes, and calcium hypochlorite.

What Harm Can They Do?

The acids in toilet bowl cleaners need to be strong to dissolve the accumulated minerals of iron, magnesium, and calcium left there from the evaporating water. The powdered toilet bowl cleaners often produce sulfuric acid when mixed with water. Sulfuric acid is highly corrosive and toxic. Even dilute sulfuric acid is a serious irritant, so take care not to breathe in the vapor from the powdered toilet bowl cleaners and guard against splashing your eyes or skin. If an acid is strong enough to dissolve mineral stains, what do you think will happen if you accidentally get a splash or two? I don't like to think about it, so I won't buy commercial toilet bowl cleaners. What manufacturers of toilet bowl cleaners don't tell you is that there is another way to remove those persistent rings without using dangerous chemicals: the wonderful pumice stone. Acidic toilet bowl cleaners are especially dangerous if mixed with bleach because they can form poisonous chlorine gas. Chemicals in toilet bowl cleaners are particularly troublesome because the toilet is one of the most common areas in the house where dangerous chemicals are combined.

Recently I was at a dinner party, sharing stories about nontoxic cleaners. A lady told me that her friend had been busily cleaning house in preparation for a dinner party for her husband's business associates. He came home from work and found her unconscious on the bathroom floor. Unaware of the potential for danger, she had mixed an acidic powdered toilet bowl cleaner with some ordinary household bleach, and toxic chlorine gas had resulted. The gas compromised her breathing enough that she became unconscious. It was off to the emergency room for her—she had severe burns in her nose and throat. Party ruined.

Note: The Poison Control Center people I've talked to said that you usually won't find someone unconscious from this kind of thing. Most people smell it and run before the gas does damage that serious. Nevertheless, this is a true story. This type of thing can happen and can result in serious lung damage. **Please do not mix the following in a toilet or anywhere: ammonia and bleach, toilet bowl cleaner and bleach, or vinegar and bleach. Dangerous gases can result.**

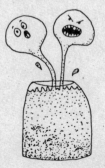

Getting Ready to Clean Nontoxically

Before you can start your toilet bowl cleaning, you need to remove any automatic toilet bowl cleaners in the toilet tank. Yes, that means check under the lid and see if

---

Hollywood Bowl
Toilet Bowl Cleaner

This recipe is really a version of my Earth Scrub™ recipe but with the added disinfecting power of tea tree oil.

Ingredients: Liquid soap or detergent, baking soda, white vinegar, tea tree oil, and water.

What Else You'll Need: A 22-oz. squirt-bottle (see p. 43 for a discussion on getting the right kind of bottle).

How to Make: Mix the ½ cup liquid soap and 2 cups baking soda together. I like to use Dr. Bronner's peppermint or euca- lyptus soap for this recipe. Work out any lumps with a fork. Dilute with ¼ cup water and add 2 tbsp. vinegar to make it foam. Add ½ teaspoon of tea tree oil (½ tsp. = 50 drops or 1 dropperful). When measuring the oil, use a *metal* measuring spoon or estimate with a dinner spoon. Don't use plastic spoons. Mix and pour the final solution into a 22-oz. squirt-bottle. Shake the bottle well before using the cleaner.

How to Use: Squirt the cleaner inside the toilet, on and under the rim, and on the seats. I use a high-quality toilet brush for the inside and a sponge for the rim and seats. Rinse with a scented vinegar if you like.

Effectiveness Rating: 100%

Commercial Brand* vs. Hollywood Bowl (24-oz. toilet bowl cleaner): $2.47 vs. $1.61. 2 cups baking soda costs about 60¢, ½ cup liquid detergent costs about 25¢, and 2 tbsp. vinegar about 2¢. You'll save 86¢ each time you refill the bottle.

---

*Price comparison with Clorox Clean Up.

an automatic cleaner is there. The amount of bleach that is dispensed from an automatic toilet bowl cleaner should not cause you a problem, but just to be safe, remove it anyway. You don't really know what's in that automatic toilet bowl cleaner, and you don't want to be mixing even your relatively safe homemade cleaners with it. Please take it out and save it for hazardous waste disposal.

Here is my number-one toilet bowl cleaning rule: *Don't use the cheap kind of toilet bowl brushes that have the twisted metal loop.* If you have one, throw it away. Those brushes cause more problems than they are worth, and they certainly don't last. The bristles aren't strong enough and quickly wear down, exposing the metal twist. When you use an old toilet brush like this, you end up scratching the porcelain with the metal, which causes the bowl to collect dirt and stains more easily. The metal also rusts, leaving stains wherever you put it. Spend a few dollars more for the kind with the tough plastic interior. They last a lot longer, work better right away, and won't scratch your toilet bowl. It's worth it!

Sleepy Head
Toilet Bowl Cleaner

Too tired and sleepy to clean your toilet bowl? Try this wonderfully lazy way to disinfect and deodorize. Easy and quick, this is one of the first cleaning recipes that I tried.

Ingredients: Borax (found in the laundry section, often in a green box) and tea tree oil (if you like).

How to Make: Add 20–30 drops of tea tree oil to ¹/₂ cup borax.

What to Do: Pour borax straight from the box into your toilet bowl. I use approximately ½ cup. Add 20–30 drops of tea tree oil. The tea tree oil adds a little disinfecting power and strong, clean smell. Next, hold the toilet brush over the bowl and sprinkle on some borax. Give the inside edges a good swish with it. Close the lid and leave the toilet overnight. While you are sleeping the borax will be busy cleaning. In the morning, swish the bowl with your toilet brush, and you are done. Sometimes I scent the borax ahead of time, but most of the time, I use it straight from the box. Add about 30 drops of tea tree oil for each cup of borax.

Effectiveness Rating: 70%

Commercial Brand* vs. Sleepy Head (automatic toilet bowl cleaner): $3.29 vs. .92¢. ½ cup borax costs 8¢, and the disinfecting scent costs 15¢. Comparing monthly applications of borax for 4 months with a tank dispenser of 2000 Flushes, which lasts 4 months, you'll **save** $2.90.

---

*Price comparison with 2000 Flushes.

A Note About Borax

Borax, a common ingredient in all fabric bleaches, is the strongest chemical cleaner that I keep around the house. Although it is reputed to have antiseptic, disinfectant, and antifungal properties, I rarely use it. I don't consider it nontoxic. Borax is a strong alkaline, an eye irritant, and toxic if swallowed. I always keep it on a shelf in the laundry room away from my toddler. I've tried using borax for cleaning, as a powder or cleanser, but it irritates my hands. I've also read warnings that you shouldn't get borax in open cuts because it is absorbed readily into the system this way. I always seem to have a small scratch or open cut on my hands, so that makes using it as a cleanser pretty impossible unless I want to wear gloves. So, I limit my uses of borax to cleaning situations where I don't have to touch it: in the laundry, in the toilet, in the garbage can, and in a bucket as a diaper soak.

What Do I Use for Cleaning the Toilet?

Honestly, I have to say I use whatever is handy to clean my toilet. That means whatever cleaner I have recently made and is under the sink in the bathroom. One of my favorites is Merlin's Magic™ antiseptic soap spray (see pp. 114–15). I use it for the toilet seat and outside porcelain first. Then, to clean the inside of the bowl, I turn the water off just as the bowl empties. (The water turn-off knob is usually right at the back of your toilet.) The bowl cleans better when it's not full of water. I like to use my Hollywood Bowl recipe for the bowl creepies. It suds up nicely, squirts right up under the rim and around the inside bowl, and smells great. I use either a toilet brush or sponge to get at those ickies under the rim. Most of us are squeamish about sticking our fingers in a toilet bowl and like to use the toilet brush. But using a sponge can be more effective. For other cleaning, I don't like to use gloves, but for cleaning toilets, using gloves makes a lot of sense. Next, I squirt the outside porcelain and rim and then wipe or brush. I finish with a scented vinegar rinse that gets off any remaining residue in the corners and edges. Finally, I dry the outside with a clean rag, turn the water back on, rinse the brush, and I'm done.

Why do we despise cleaning a toilet so? Mostly because we have been taught that it is really yucky even though the constant flow of water in the bowl keeps it relatively clean. Surprisingly enough, the really dirty part of the toilet is the base (where old urine spills ferment), underneath the seat (more backsplash), and under the rim (where ye olde molds love to grow). You can use several different recipes of mine for the seat covers and outside base, such as Alice's Wonder Spray™ (see pp. 85–86), Momma's Earth Mop™ (see pp. 135–36), Merlin's Magic™ (see pp. 114–15), Hollywood Bowl (see p. 230), Earth Scrub™ (see pp. 239–40), or EarthShaker™ (see pp. 185–86). A spray-bottle is great for the toilet because it gets at all the corners, crevices, and curves, but a squirter works quite well, too. Using a scented vinegar will also eliminate any urine smell that may be sticking around. Be sure to use it at the base, especially if you have carpet in your bathroom! When you're finished, if you want to make sure the toilet bowl brush is really disinfected, then put your brush and brush holder in the bathtub. Sprinkle some salt on the brush, fill the brush caddy with hot water, swish, and let it sit for 5 minutes or more. The salty water will help to disinfect it.

What to Use on Yellow, Stained, and Icky Toilet Bowls

If your toilet is badly stained, start with the Sleepy Head recipe of tea tree oil–scented borax. An overnight soak with borax has freshened up many a dreary bowl. In the morning, just rub with a toilet brush and flush. Next, you'll need your gloves and the most powerhouse nontoxic toilet bowl cleaner of all, the pumice stone. It's a fantastic and effective alternative to those dangerous toilet bowl cleaners. With the inexpensive, nontoxic pumice stone, I've gotten out stains from toilets that hadn't been cleaned for 3 or 4 years! You'll want to get a glove on, wet your stone (I let mine just sit in the bowl for 1 or 2 minutes), and then start rubbing. The stone makes a loud scratching sound but swiftly gets those nasty stains away. Keep rubbing, and they will all be gone. Before I tried it, I was convinced the pumice stone would scratch. Don't worry! Your porcelain is harder than your pumice stone. As long as you keep the stone wet, you will have no problem. It's really hardly a stone anyway; it's more like a soft sand that sticks together. It's good for cleaning nasty spots in an oven, too. Please, try this wonder stone and don't resort to those nasty acids. They make a mess of the environment and are a danger to have in the house.

A boy I met in college told me that he actually fell in love with me as he watched me cleaning a toilet. We are still friends today. You see, toilet bowl cleaning isn't that bad after all.

Tub and Tile Cleaners

What's Really in Them?

Ingredients in tub and tile cleaners include sodium hypochlorite (bleach), sodium hydroxide (lye), phosphoric acid, ammonia, ethanol, and detergents.

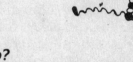

What Harm Can They Do?

When inhaled, they can dissolve and damage your delicate lung tissue much in the same way that they dissolve tenacious mildew or soap film. The ammonia and ethanols can also be irritating to the lungs. You should avoid them especially if you or your children have respiratory problems such as asthma or bronchitis. Small children, older people, and those with even mild respiratory problems or heart conditions are better off not breathing any product that contains any ammonia, bleach, or lye. I think it's even true to say that we are *all* better off not breathing any of those chemicals!

"What's the cleaner you dislike using the most?" I asked my cleaning-professional friends. Their responses: "Tilex. It smells terrible."; "Tilex. It make me sick."; "I always get headaches when I use Tilex or X-14 to clean the shower." Their answers were always the same. Even toilet bowl cleaners and drain cleaners rate better because they don't have to breathe them as much. Is it really safe to have this type of product on the market? Especially in an aerosol? The reality is that when you are cleaning a tub and shower you can't help but *inhale deeply* whatever you are cleaning with. I was rinsing a tub and shower with a peppermint-scented vinegar the other day. I leaned over, and pow, the peppermint scent hit me. It was great scent and made me feel good. How horrible it would be if I were cleaning with something toxic and damaging to my lungs. Tub and showers are enclosed spaces that concentrate the vapors of whatever you are using to clean it. Manufacturers of these cleaners put a warning on the label to ventilate the area when using, but opening a window rarely adequately ventilates an enclosed tub or shower. Efforts to properly ventilate these areas, such as moving a fan around the house to air out the bathrooms as you clean, are impractical suggestions and, in real life, almost never done.

Cleaning super mildew problems can be tough. Investing in a couple of professional-quality tile and cleaning toothbrushes is a nontoxic choice (see Cleaning Catalogs in the Resources section). Add some Bon Ami cleanser and determination, and you have the problem solved. But the very best suggestion is to prevent them. Here are four wise ways to prevent mildew in the bathroom:

1. *Mildew will not grow in dry air and sunlight.* If you have a mildew problem, then keeping that window

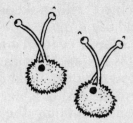

and/or door open when you are taking a hot shower makes a lot of sense. Try putting on the fan more often. Or if you don't already have one, install a new one or get a small countertop fan. Letting steam and water sit on walls, showers, and floors only invites trouble. Wallpapers peel, corners start to grow things, glues loosen, floors curl, grout turns green, and you can get a case of the tenacious mildew blues. If you are a "cold" ninny like me, you can keep the door closed during the shower, but open it as soon as you have toweled dry. And let the sun come in. If you're stuck with an unavoidably "dark" bathroom, then even leaving the lights on for a while after your shower can help to retard mildew growth.

2. *Oil resists water.* Moisture, water, and lack of light cause mildew to grow. Wiping down mildew-prone areas with an oily rag can help the moisture to stay away. Or try a vinegar rinse a couple of times a week to see if the mildew stays away.

3. *Use a squeegee to wipe down your walls after the shower.* This suggestion really works! Taking the moisture directly off your shower walls keeps the mold and mildew from forming and sends that clingy soap film down the drain. I keep a small, yellow (6-in.) squeegee handy in a bucket by the shower with the sliding glass doors just for this very purpose. A regular window-washing size squeegee is too big and ugly. My daughter loves to pretend to window-wash with the small one, too. We only use it occasionally, but if we

had a serious problem with mold or mildew build-up, I'm sure we would use it more.

4. *Use only a cloth shower curtain and forget about the plastic liner on the inside.* My plastic shower curtain would always grow mildew, making it unpleasant to take a shower, embarrassing when I had guests, and annoying to clean. Scrubbing the bottom of a mildewed $4.25 plastic shower curtain for 20 minutes is not the way I want to spend my Saturday morning. Keeping the shower curtain pulled closed to its full width helped some, but the mildew kept coming anyway. Someone told me that I could throw that curtain right into the washer with a couple of towels and easily remove the beginning stages of mildew. That tip worked great. The mildew came out, but . . . it was a pain to unhook and rehook that curtain every time I wanted to wash it. What to do? Well, one day after washing that plastic shower curtain, I folded it up and just didn't hang it back up. I had an outside cloth shower curtain cover and just started using that. I pull the cloth curtain into the tub for the shower, squeeze it dry before I pull it out after the shower, and try to keep it closed to its full width during the day. But that's about it. Most cloth shower curtains work just fine without an inside plastic liner. Since it's cloth, it dries quicker than the plastic kind. We've never had a spot of mildew since.

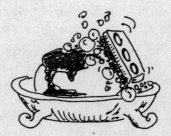

Earth Scrub™
Tub and Tile Cleaner

For most everyday tub and tile cleaning, you really need only a simple, pleasant cleaner. Have I got a recipe for you . . . your own homemade Soft Scrub alternative!

Ingredients: Baking soda, a high-quality liquid soap, white distilled vinegar, and water.

What Else You'll Need: A 16-oz. squeeze container with a special kind of squirt flip-top cap. Only a few types of squirt-tops will work for this recipe (see Getting the Right Container for Earth Scrub™, p. 240). Otherwise, they clog.

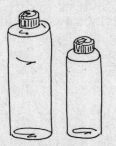

22- or 16-oz. flip-top bottles

How to Make: *For a 16-oz. bottle:* Mix 1⅔ cups baking soda with ½ cup of liquid soap in a bowl. (I highly suggest using liquid soaps for this recipe because if you use liquid detergents, it makes this scrub too time consuming to rinse off.) Dilute with ½ cup water. Add the 2 tbsp. vinegar *last*. Stir until the lumps are gone. If you can pour it into the container easily, then you have the right consistency. If it's too thick, add more water. Keep the cap on, because this mixture will dry out. Shake well before using. *For a 22-oz. bottle:* Mix 2 cups baking soda, ½ cup liquid soap, ⅔ cup water, and 2 tbsp. vinegar (add the vinegar *last*).

How to Use: Squirt this excellent cleaner anywhere! My favorite places to use it are the tub, sink, and toilet bowl, but I've used it for floors, garbage cans, and any greasy, grimy job.

It's also great for under the rim of the toilet, bathtub rings, sinks, and countertops. It's an absolutely *soft*, mildly abrasive cleanser. Use it with a nylon white-backed sponge to prevent scratching. Rinse well. If you find that you are leaving a baking-soda residue (a white dust after it dries), try using a little less scrub next time and/or rinse with a squirt of scented vinegar and water. A vinegar rinse may help to prevent mold and mildew, too. In this cleaner, the baking soda and soap will tend to separate, so make sure to *shake well before using*. Measure this recipe carefully. Be as exact as you can; otherwise, your squirt will be too thin or thick. Mix the baking soda and soap together well with a fork, and *add that vinegar last*.

Effectiveness Rating: 90%–100%

Commercial Brand* vs. Earth Scrub™ (26-oz. tub and tile cleaner): $3.27 vs. $1.61. 2 cups baking soda costs about 60¢, ½ cup liquid soap costs you about 99¢, and 2 tbsp. vinegar costs about 2¢. You'll **save** $1.66 each time you refill the bottle.

---

*Price comparison with Soft Scrub.

Getting the Right Container for Earth Scrub™

Earth Scrub™ is such a terrific recipe it's worth the extra hassle trying to find the right container for it. Most shampoo-type bottles have squirt tops that clog. For use with this recipe, here are three ways to get one that works:

1. *Reuse the Soft Scrub bottle top* with a clean, new 16- or 22-oz. squeeze bottle. It's a great top but notice that I said to reuse only the bottle top, not the whole bottle. Rinse the bottle top out thoroughly before reusing. The hole will clog up occasionally. All you have to do is poke it with a pen or pencil or rub it with your finger on the underside, and it's working again.
2. *You can get a bottle from me.* I found the special kind of bottle top with the right-size hole that works best

and clogs the least. You can get a 16-oz. squeeze bottle and a pretty label with the Earth Scrub™ recipe right on it. It's very similar to the top of a Soft Scrub bottle and works just about the same.

3. *You can buy a Rubbermaid Servin' Saver Squeeze and Squirt bottle in the grocery store.* This container works well, but it's expensive and dispenses more than I would like. On the brighter side, this bottle has a large lid that makes it easy to fill the bottle and stir the cleaner. This bottle squeezes nicely.

Getting the Right Baking Soda for Earth Scrub™

I highly suggest that you buy the Arm & Hammer baking soda for this recipe. In this case, the expensive brand is the superior one. Buying Arm & Hammer baking soda is well worth the price, especially for the tub-and-tile cleaner recipes. Arm & Hammer mixes well with other ingredients, retains the scents longer, and makes a more smooth cleaner. Compare it with the generic baking soda yourself. The Arm & Hammer's particle size is finer and seems to clump up less. The generic baking soda I kept under my kitchen sink clumped. Clumps are a hassle when you're mixing up recipes. Spend a few more pennies for quality.

Tackling Slimy Soap Film

How do you get rid of that soap film in the tub or shower? *Scrub!* I use a handled scrubber that I got from the Clean Team catalog (see Resources section, p. 285). If you are tackling months' or years' worth of soap build-up, you will need a power tool like Clean Team's Grab & Scrub. You'll also need some vinegar because the scrubber gets clogged with soap build-up. Fill the sink with an inch or so of vinegar and drop the scrubber in every once in a while to dissolve the soap. Squirting the walls with vinegar and letting it sit helps a little bit, but if you are looking at a thick white soap-film build-up from months and months of zero cleaning, don't expect much of a result. Vinegar cuts a *thin* soap film but won't cut months' or years' worth of build-up. Your best bet is to use the scrubber, or, if it's *really* thick, use very fine steel wool to get off the first layer. Use that steel wool gently, though!

Build-up Prevention

Here are three easy ways to prevent soap build-up in the bathroom:

1. *While you are taking a shower, take a little time out to scrub away the soap ring in the tub and then take a quick swipe at the shower walls and doors.* I keep a bottle of Earth Scrub™ on the ledge with the shampoo bottles just for this very purpose. Or just dab your sponge in your baking-soda deodorizer box (see Good Clean Scents, p. 72) on the top of the toilet and scrub. Rinse with a scented vinegar. Cleaning opportunities are everywhere. Now that you have nontoxics, you can start enjoying them.
2. *At the end of any shower, squirt-clean your shower walls once or twice a week with your favorite scented vinegar recipe.* I also keep a small bottle of scented vinegar on the shampoo bottle ledge for that purpose. Squirting a scented vinegar on your walls is fun and may help to prevent mold and mildew; you don't even have to rinse it!
3. *Use that squeegee—the one you use to prevent mildew—to wipe away the soap and water drips on the wall.* It's the dissolved soap drying on the walls that makes the soap build-up. With a cute little 6-in. squeegee, you can send that soap film down the drain.

Earth Paste™
Tub and Tile Cleaner

Earth Paste™ is easy to make and, by anyone's standard, a delightful bathroom cleaner. It's almost identical to the Earth Scrub™ recipe (see pp. 239–40) except that it's a thicker scrub and you can store it in a jar. I like to use Dr. Bronner's almond-scented liquid soap for this recipe. When I make this recipe, it reminds me of butter cream frosting, making the mixture seem awfully edible. But, please, don't eat it! Remember, it's soap, after all.

Ingredients: Baking soda, liquid soap, white distilled vinegar, and water.

What Else You'll Need: A clean 16-oz. plastic or glass wide-mouthed jar. Most jars do not seal tightly enough to keep this recipe fresh. Only a few types of jars work (see Getting the Right Jar for Earth Paste™, p. 244).

How to Make: Mix 1 2/3 cup baking soda with 1/2 cup liquid soap in a bowl. (I highly suggest using liquid soaps for this recipe because I've found that liquid detergents are too time consuming to rinse off). Add 2 tbsp. water. Mix with a fork until smooth. Stir in 2 tbsp. vinegar *last*. The mixture will foam nicely. Use a spatula to scoop your homemade scrub into the jar. Store this mixture in a plastic or glass jar. Add warm water if the paste dries out. You may need to stir this recipe a little before using. *When mixing this paste, don't mix the vinegar and the soap directly together or you will make gunk instead of scrub.* Add the vinegar *last*.

How to Use: Scoop this fragrant, enjoyable scrub right out of the jar with a soft cloth or sponge and start cleaning. Rinse well. If you find you are leaving baking-soda residue, use a scented vinegar to rinse and your tubs will be squeaky clean! As you squirt the vinegar, you'll hear a tiny fizz. That's just the baking soda and vinegar mixing to form a bit of harmless carbon dioxide gas. The fizzing actually makes it fun. If the jar top is not tight enough, the scrub will dry out eventually. If your scrub dries out, then add a little water and let it sit to help the baking soda soften, then mix with a fork. See my suggestions for getting the right jar.

Effectiveness Rating: 90%–100%

Commercial Brand* vs. Earth Paste™ (17-oz. tub and tile cleaner): $2.79 vs. $1.12. 2 cups baking soda costs about 60¢, ½ cup liquid soap costs about 50¢, and 2 tbsp. vinegar costs about 2¢. You'll **save** $1.67.

*Price comparison with Scrubbing Bubbles (by Dow Chemical Company).

Getting the Right Jar for Earth Paste™

Most jars are not tight enough to keep your Earth Paste™ from drying out for very long. Here are a few options:

1. *Put a cut-up soggy sponge in the jar.* The easiest way to make any jar work is to cut up a small piece of an old sponge, soak it in water, and put it inside the jar. The soggy sponge will help to keep that paste moist for at least several months. Rewet the sponge as necessary. **Important:** *If you are reusing a jar, be sure to remove the old label and put on a new label. You don't want anyone mistaking your recipe for food or other items.* Mark the label clearly as Earth Paste™ with the ingredients of baking soda, soap, and vinegar. To make it last, laminate that label with the plastic sheets you can get from an office-supply store.
2. *Use a tightly sealed jar.* This idea may not sound appealing, but it works great. If you are a brand-new mom, you may have a jar of Tufts hemorrhoidal pads in the house. This is the perfect type of jar. If you do reuse it, it's important to make sure to remove the old label and put on a new label. Remember to mark it clearly as Earth Paste™ with the ingredients of baking soda, soap, and vinegar.
3. *You can order a jar from me.* I found a jar that seals so nicely that the recipe will never dry out! It comes with the Earth Paste™ recipe right on the label.

4. *Make up only what you need at any one time.* Lots of times, I make up only a small bowl of Earth Paste™ and use it for cleaning the tub, toilet, and sinks. If there's a little bit left over, I use it the next day for hand-washing the dishes or kitchen sink.

Many people I know use a simple powder cleanser to clean their bathtub. Powdered cleansers are often much less expensive than almost any other type of bathroom cleaner. Watch out, though; some can scratch. I've used my EarthShaker™ recipe of scented baking soda right from the kitchen sink instead. It's so nontoxic that I can let my daughter play with it while I clean the tub. But don't leave behind piles of baking soda to sit on your tub edges. It can roughen delicate surfaces if left on long enough. Here's the cost comparison to one of those fancier bathroom cleaning gels:

Commercial Brand* vs. EarthShaker™ (22-oz. tub and tile cleaner): **$2.79 vs. 77¢.** 2½ cups baking soda costs about 50¢. A nice scent costs about 22¢. You'll **save** $2.02.

*Price comparison with Clorox Clean Up.

Homemade recipes with a personal touch make great gifts. Make up your own name and personalize the scent and label. Here's an example of one of my favorite ways to scent and give away an Earth Paste™.

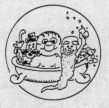

Baby Elephant Scrub

Whenever I make this recipe, I like it so much that I can't resist trying it out immediately on the tub. I use Dr. Bronner's baby castile soap and a squirt of strawberry oil. It's a fun scrub for which you'll want to design your own personalized label so you can give it to someone as a gift.

Ingredients: Baking soda, liquid soap, white distilled vinegar, and water.

What Else You'll Need: An 8-oz. jar.

How to Make: In a jar or bowl, mix 1 cup baking soda with 1/4 cup unscented liquid soap. Work out the clumps with a fork. Add 1 tbsp. white vinegar and stir. Use a spatula to spoon your mixture into the jar. Now add your scent. I use 25 drops of strawberry oil (equivalent to 1/4 tsp. or 1/2 dropperful). Another favorite scent of mine is a mixture of apple (15 drops) and peach (20 drops) oils. Add a drop or two of red food coloring and you'll have pink elephant scrub, too!

How to Use: Use as you would any Earth Scrub™. If you are giving this away as a gift, make sure to get a jar that seals tightly so the scrub doesn't dry out. Don't forget to laminate the label and list all the ingredients, including the fragrance. And be sure to include the warnings for any soap: don't eat, and keep out of eyes.

Your Tender Tub and Tile

Most tubs are Fiberglas these days and need to be treated gently. Anything abrasive will dull and scratch the surface, making it more difficult to clean the next time around. When you clean, use only the softest cleaners with a rag or nylon white-backed sponge. No green-backed sponges, please.

Please don't use your tubs as chemical garbage disposals. Chemicals can damage the finish on your tub or leave hazardous residues. Store those chemicals in a safe place and take them to a hazardous waste disposal center. Please, don't ever dump paint thinner, paint, varnishes, or the like down the toilet, tub, or drain. These types of chemicals ruin the effectiveness of wastewater treatment. In my city, it's actually illegal to put those items down the drain.

Be careful with the marble, please! Marble in the bathroom is beautiful, but it's delicate. An extremely soft stone, marble can stain and scratch quite easily. Many manufacturers recommend using mild soap and water only. If you do need to use a stronger cleanser, you can use a little Earth Scrub™, but be gentle. Baking soda is mildly abrasive. It dissolves quickly with water, but to make sure every bit of it is gone, you should rinse with a diluted scented vinegar. Even a slight baking-soda residue left on too long could roughen your marble's delicate surface.

Scented Baking Sodas

Scented Baking Sodas

Making your own scented baking sodas is fun and inexpensive. Here are the basic instructions and measurements for scenting your own. Once you've tried a few, you'll be hooked!

Ingredients: Baking soda and essential oils.

What Else You'll Need: A fork.

How to Make: I usually scent my baking sodas right in the box. I open the top part of the cardboard box and carefully pull it all the way back, poke little holes in the soda with my fingers, and then drop in the oils. Don't put the pools of oil too close to the side of the box or the cardboard will just wick it up. Mix the oil into the baking soda with a fork. I dig into one side and then the other side for a thorough mixing. You don't have to get to the bottom completely because the odor will generally dissipate into the entire box. If you have asthma or other respiratory problems, mix very gently or just push the oil into the soda. Anything particulate will irritate the lungs. **I wish they sold a pure essential oil–scented baking soda in the supermarket, but they don't yet!** After I've mixed in the oil, I re-cover the box with the top and tape it shut with masking tape so that I still have a convenient pour spout on the side with which to fill my shakers. I keep my masking tape in the junk drawer in the kitchen, essential oils in with the spices, and the baking soda boxes under the sink. So I'm always ready to make up a new batch.

How I measure in the oils depends on what kind of essential-oil bottle I have. I use either drops, a glass dropper, or a metal teaspoon. Using a glass dropper is the quickest, but you have to buy the empty bottle with the dropper separately and fill it with the oil yourself. Oils aren't sold with droppers because over time, the aroma of the oil can dissolve the plastic bulb at the top of the dropper. You will probably find using the small bottles with a plastic dropper spout already built into the bottle to be the most convenient. Many of the oils you can purchase are sold this way, but it takes some patience to count up to 50 drops or so. If you lose count, don't worry; you don't have to be exact. Just scent the soda as you like.

Be careful when using the oils. Oils are very powerful and concentrated and can irritate the skin. I keep a rag handy to pick up any spills or drips on the bottles. Some essential oils are dangerously toxic so I'd stick with the oils I suggest. Because they are concentrated, all oils need to be kept out of the reach of children. Check with your essential-oil company if you have a question. I use lemon, peppermint, and tea tree oils the most. Lavender oils can vary in quality, so I tend to avoid them. If you find a good one, stick with it. Although synthetic oils can be irritating to those with sensitivities, I still use apple, strawberry, and rose fragrances occasionally.

Essential oils can vary in strength, so here are the measurements for a few of my favorite scents.

Lemon Lovers
Lemon-Scented Baking Soda

Lemon is one of my favorite cleaning scents because lemons are naturally great cleaners. Lemon oil adds extra cleaning power to your soda and a pungent freshness every time you scrub. Add a little lime, too, if you like.

Ingredients: Lemon and/or lime pure essential oils. Ask for food-grade pure essential oils; don't accept a synthetic substitute.

To Scent: For a 2-lb. box, add 50 drops of lemon oil (50 drops = 1 dropperful or ½ tsp.). Add an equal amount of lime oil, if you like. Double these measurements for a 4-lb. box.

Sweet Memories
Lavender-Scented Baking Soda

This is a delightful, sweet, floral scent to have under your kitchen or bathroom sink.

Ingredients: Pure essential lavender oil.

To Scent: For a 2-lb. box, add 10 drops of lavender oil (10 drops = ⅕ dropperful or ⅛ tsp.). Double this measurement for a 4-lb. box.

Forever Strawberry
Scented Baking Soda

Almost too delicious of a scent to use for a cleaner, a strawberry scent is the unanimous favorite for kids. I put this soda in a decorative box in the bathroom as an air freshener.

Ingredients: Strawberry oil (always a synthetic fragrance).

To Scent: For a 2-lb. box, add 35 drops of strawberry oil (35 drops = ¾ dropperful or ½ tsp.). Double these measurements for a 4-lb. box.

Peppermint Pick-Me-Up
Scented Baking Soda

Using a peppermint-scented baking soda at your sink helps you to wake up in the morning and stay alert at night when you are finishing up the last of those dinner dishes. Try it. It's also a great emergency toothpaste! If you do use it for toothpaste, be sure to get the food-grade–quality pure essential peppermint oil. Don't use too much oil just to get a taste! Every essential oil is very powerful and needs to be diluted for use.

Ingredients: Peppermint oil (ask for food-grade–quality pure essential oil).

To Scent: For a 2-lb. box, add 25 drops of peppermint oil (25 drops = ½ dropperful or ¼ tsp.). Double these measurements for a 4-lb. box.

Miniature Roses
Scented Baking Soda

This is the most subtle of all the baking-soda scents. I've fresh-ened up musty clothes by sprinkling on this delightful rose baking soda, letting them sit for a couple of hours to help de-odorize, and then washing them. This is a perfect scent for a birthday or baby-shower gift.

Ingredients: Rose oil. You can get a pure rose oil, but it's very expensive. The kind you can afford is always synthetic. If you want to go natural less expensively, grind up your own rose petals and add to the baking soda. The particles of rose petals are a bit annoying to clean with, but in a box it makes a subtle, delightful air freshener.

To Scent: For a 2-lb. box, add 25 drops of rose oil (25 drops = $\frac{1}{2}$ dropperful or $\frac{1}{4}$ tsp.). Double these measure-ments for a 4-lb. box.

Peachy Clean
Scented Baking Soda

This is a very refined scent for a baking-soda cleaner. You might be disappointed with this fragrance because it's not very strong. If you have a sensitive sniffer, though, you'll love its soft, sweet scent.

Ingredients: Peach oil (a very subtle, synthetic fragrance).

To Scent: For a 2-lb. box, add 25 drops of peach oil (25 drops = $\frac{1}{2}$ dropperful or $\frac{1}{4}$ tsp.). Double these measure-ments for a 4-lb. box.

Tea-rrific Tea Tree
Scented Baking Soda

Using the wonder oil from Australia, tea tree oil, makes for a great scented baking soda for cleaning and deodorizing the toilet and the diaper pail. If you don't already know about this antifungal, antibacterial oil, go to your local health-food store and ask about it. It has so many wonderful uses.

Ingredients: Tea tree oil (ask for a pure essential one, such as the one sold under the Desert Essence label).

To Scent: For a 2-lb. box, add 25 drops of tea tree oil (25 drops = ½ dropperful or ¼ tsp.). Double these measurements for a 4-lb. box.

Scented Vinegars

I like to clean with vinegar, but I hate the smell. To solve the problem, I give that vinegar my own homemade scent by adding pure essential oils and fragrances. Most white distilled vinegars come in gallon jugs. It's easy and quick to scent them right in the jug, and the fragrances last long enough for general use. Always use the *white* distilled vinegar, and buy the Heinz brand if you can; I think it smells better than other brands' vinegars. Other vinegars can be made from petroleum, but Heinz is made from corn. I buy mine in large quantities at a discount house.

To make scenting your vinegars easy, I've measured the essential oils in three different ways: with a teaspoon, with a dropper, or as drops. Test the strength of the scent by pouring a little vinegar on a sponge, wiping the counter, and sniffing. It's too strong to sniff directly from the jug. As always, be careful with the essential oils. They are concentrated and can dissolve plastics when spilled.

Peppy Mint Vinegar
Scented Vinegar

This is a fun, happy, zippy scent to clean with and my favorite scent for a floor cleaner.

Ingredients: Peppermint oil and white distilled vinegar.

To scent 1 gallon of vinegar: Use 50 drops of peppermint oil (*or* 1 dropperful *or* 1/2 tsp.).

Apple Orchard Vinegar
Scented Vinegar

Apple is a fresh, sweet, soft fragrance to add to your vinegar. The apple really covers up that biting vinegar odor. Even though it is a synthetic fragrance, it is one of my favorite vinegar scents. Don't use too much—a little goes a long way. If you are sensitive to perfume smells, you probably won't like this one. I often use this sweet-scented vinegar as a laundry rinse.

Ingredients: Apple fragrance oil and white distilled vinegar.

To scent 1 gallon of vinegar: Use 25 drops of apple fragrance (*or* 1/2 dropperful *or* 1/4 tsp.).

Sniff-It Eucalyptus Vinegar

Scented Vinegar

This is great for clearing your nose, and the eucalyptus scent in this vinegar will leave the room you cleaned smelling fragrant and fresh.

Ingredients: Eucalyptus oil and white distilled vinegar.

To scent 1 gallon of vinegar: Use 50 drops of eucalyptus oil (*or* 1 dropperful *or* 1/2 tsp.).

Love That Lavender Vinegar

Scented Vinegar

Some people like it; some people don't. It's sure to bring back memories of Grandma's house or a hand-me-down flowery quilt. Apparently, there are more than 160 varieties of lavender flowers.

Ingredients: Lavender oil and white distilled vinegar.

To scent 1 gallon of vinegar: Use 75 drops of lavender oil (*or* 1 1/2 dropperfuls *or* 3/4 tsp.).

Australian Tree Vinegar

Scented Vinegar

Adding tea tree oil to your vinegar gives it disinfecting power and a powerful antiseptic fragrance. I use this vinegar when I need a large quantity of disinfectant and/or deodorizer for walls, floors, or shower curtains. Both vinegar and tea tree oil are supposed to help to prevent mold and mildew.

Ingredients: Tea tree oil and white distilled vinegar.

To scent 1 gallon of vinegar: Use 75 drops of tea tree oil (*or* 1 ½ dropperfuls *or* ¾ tsp.).

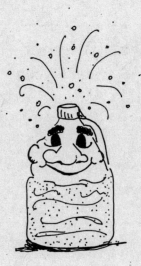

P·A·R·T VI

Cleaning Questions and Answers

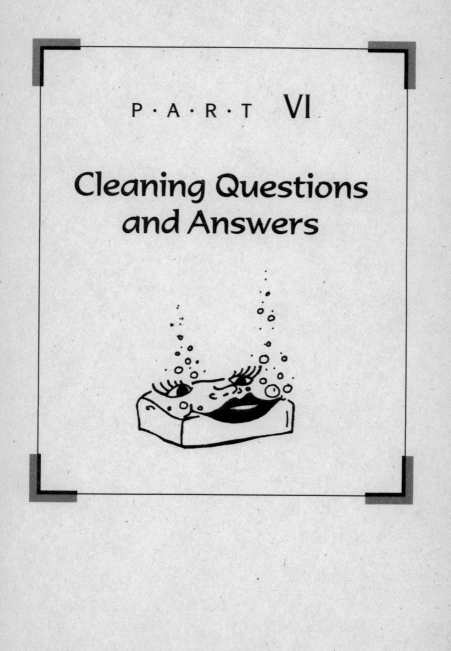

Where Do You Get Essential Oils?

You can get essential oils from your local health-food store or by mail order. Be sure to ask for pure essential oil, the kind made from the actual fruit, flower, or plant. I also use apple and strawberry fragrances in some recipes, but these are not essential oils. Fragrances are synthetic and can irritate those with sensitivities. The most environmentally kind choice is a pure organic essential oil such as lemon, lime, peppermint, lavender, eucalyptus, or tea tree. I order my fragrances and oils by mail from Frontier Herbs:

> Frontier Herbs (catalog company)
> 2264 Market Street
> San Francisco, CA 94114
> (800) 786-1388
> (415) 621-8444

Tell the person answering the phone that you want to buy retail; otherwise, he or she may assume you are a wholesale buyer. I'd start with just a few of the ⅓-oz. bottles of peppermint, lemon, lavender, and tea tree oils. They also offer certified organic essential oils. Prices for ⅓ oz. of essential oils generally range from $5 to $10 each. They also sell Aura Cacia brand oils that are sometimes a little less expensive and come in ½-oz. bottles. If you make a lot of cleaning products like I do, you'll want to get the larger 4-oz. bottles. *I buy an empty 1⅓-oz. bottle and refill it from my 4-oz. bottle. Be sure to order a dropper for the 1⅓-oz. bottle; they come separately.* Droppers are a lot faster way to measure out the oils.

An important practical note: Many of the smaller essential oil bottles come with a plastic dropper spout in the top of the bottle. Tip the bottle over and wait until the oil drips out. Don't shake; it doesn't help. Have patience; turn the bottle upside down, wait a few seconds, and the oil will start dripping. If your bottle is not dripping at all, then it is defective and Frontier Herbs will gladly send you a new one.

◆

What Kind of Liquid Soap Should Be Used for These Recipes?

What kind of liquid soap should be used in my recipes? *Dr. Bronner's, Dr. Bronner's, and Dr. Bronner's.* Why am I so sold on one particular brand? Maybe it's the label that is full of Dr. Bronner's eclectic wisdom on the unity of mankind: "All One God Faith." Maybe it's the fact that the 7 million bottles of soap they sell a year are all hand-packaged. Maybe it's because they spend about 10% of the company's profits on purchasing rain forest land, shelters for the homeless, or school buses for Boys and Girls Clubs. Dr. Bronner and his sons are wonderful people and very interested in making the world a better place.

Last but not least, his soaps are terrific. They come with the doctor's personal guarantee: "The mildest, most pleasant soap you ever used or your money back!" Having learned the art of soap making from his father in Germany in the 1920s, he has good reason to offer that guarantee. The soaps are a step above any other liquid soap that I tested. Smooth and refined, they mix well with other ingredients and rinse off easily. Best of all, these soaps come in the most delightful scents. Most people go crazy over the peppermint soap. *The peppermint scent is even reputed to enhance alertness and increase performance.* A study from the University of Cincinnati found that students performed better during tests after sniffing peppermint than after no scent at all.* "The fragrance effect was about the same as low-dose caffeinated beverages," said William Dember, Ph.D., a professor of psychology at the university. Peppermint, a natural high? Why not? The soaps also come in three other scents—almond, eucalyptus, and soft lavender—and you can also get them in a pure, supermild, unscented form. I was recently delighted to find Dr. Bronner's soaps available in my local supermarket in the health-food section. Otherwise, you are sure to find them at your local health-food store.

Those of us who know Dr. Bronner from the '60s and '70s consider him to be somewhat of a legend, a rare individual who spoke out for spirituality and oneness when very few did. I had the good fortune to be able to speak with him in person at his home in Escondido, California. Although he is bedridden at the age of 87 and fragile from Parkinson's disease, his mind is still bright and alert. When I told him that I was writing a book called *Clean House, Clean Planet,* he paused, then in a whispered voice said, "It needs a third thing . . . *Clean House, Clean Planet, Clean Soul.*" He's right.

For First-Time Dr. Bronner's Users

When I was first introduced to this soap, I squeezed it on everything. Don't. It is a very mild soap, but it comes very concentrated. I use diluted Dr. Bronner's in a spray-

---

*Dember, William N., Joel S. Warm, and Raja Parasuraman. "Effects of Olfactory Stimulation on Performance and Stress in a Visual Sustained Attention Task." *The Journal of the Society of Cosmetic Chemists,* 42, p. 199–210, May/June 1991.

bottle as a quick hand wash for my toddler, counter clean-up, or handy refrigerator wipe. For use in the shower, just a few drops on a wet washcloth will do. The peppermint soap actually tingles. Write or call:

All-One-God-Faith
Rabbi Dr. E. H. Bronner Associates, SMMC
P.O. Box 28
Escondido, CA 92033
(619) 747-2211

If you don't have a health-food store nearby, you can also mail-order the soaps from The Magic Chain at (800) 622-6648.

◆

What Liquid Detergents Should Be Used for These Recipes?

For detergents, I suggest using Palmolive or Ivory liquids. I use Palmolive for sensitive skin; it has no alcohol and no dyes, and the bottle is 50% recycled plastic (unfortunately, not postconsumer waste but plastic scraps). Ivory is also good but doesn't perform quite as well. Most hand-dishwashing detergents are biodegradable and, when run through our wastewater system, have very little environmental impact at all. I wouldn't use them if I was running my dishwater into my garden, though. Ultimately, true soaps are better for the environment.

Liquid Detergents vs. Liquid Soaps

In every recipe, I've told you whether you should use a liquid soap or a liquid detergent. In a few, you do have a choice. *Detergents are usually made from petroleum*—ugh, more polluting petroleum. *True liquid castile soaps are made from vegetable oils,* a nice, renewable resource. Vegetables are pleasant to be around and less polluting than petroleum. I'm for the green. Which business would you rather support: a coconut plantation, a cattle and pig slaughterhouse, or an oil refinery? Most people would choose the coconut plantation, and for good reasons. What you don't realize is that you are making that very same choice when you decide what kind of soaps to buy for your cleaning. When you buy a detergent or any other petroleum-based product, you are voting for the oil refinery. When you buy a soap made with animal fat (such as Ivory bar soap), you are voting for the slaughterhouse. When you buy a castile soap made with vegetable oils (most commonly, coconut oil), you support the growth of more coconut plantations in the world. Coconuts are a renewable, life-supporting resource. An oil refinery operates at a huge environmental cost to air, land, and water. It's your choice.

You may think you can't afford to buy those "fancy" soaps in the health-food stores, but perhaps we can't afford not to. It's our world. We are all responsible for its health and beauty or ugliness. But you're right: liquid castile soaps are about twice as expensive as the liquid detergents you can buy in the store. Nevertheless, you will still *save* lots of money if you make my recipes with the true liquid soaps. *Go ahead and get a high-quality soap that is good for you and the environment—now you have no reason not to.*

One More Reason to Use Liquid Soaps Instead of Detergents

Squirt a little hand-dishwashing detergent into your bathroom sink. Count the number of times it takes to rinse. Now, squirt in a little Dr. Bronner's liquid soap. Count the number of times to rinse *that* away. *Detergents suds up nicely but take five to 10 times more rinsing, wasting your water and your time.* Except for my spot remover, I always use *real* liquid soaps for my cleaning recipes. If you have extremely hard water, you might find that the liquid detergents just work better. Well, then, please use them. They are great, inexpensive cleaners after all.

Here's another test. Put a small squeeze of your liquid hand-dishwashing detergent on a rag and smear it on the left side of your bathroom mirror. On the other side of your rag, squeeze a little Dr. Bronner's liquid soap and smear it on the right side of the mirror. Tell your family that you are testing a new antifog treatment. It's true: the next time you take a shower, your mirrors will not fog up. Your family and friends will be amazed, but only temporarily. Once the steam is gone, the mirrors will look disappointingly hazy with soap film. Keep your experiment on the mirrors for a couple of days. You will start to notice that the soap is streaking and dissolving from the steam water and the detergent is still a sticky film. I know I don't want that sticky detergent film left after cleaning, and I wouldn't want that detergent film floating on a local pond, either. Okay, we're finished. Clean up that hazy mirror with a squirt of vinegar and water and you're done.

Beware of those liquid soap imposters! Many products labeled as soaps on your grocery-store shelves are really liquid detergents. Companies like to use the word *soap* because it is friendlier to consumers. Here are a few examples:

- Ivory dishwashing liquid used to be a soap, but it was changed to a detergent in 1991. Liquid Ivory soap for hands contains very little real soap and mostly detergent. Its formulation was also changed in 1991.

- Softsoap and Dial for Kids and most other "antibacterial soaps" are detergents.
- Dove dishwashing liquid looks like the original white soap formulation, but it's not. It's a detergent.

Most real liquid soaps can only be found in health-food stores under brands such as: Auro Organics Natural Plant Chemistry, Biofa, Cal Ben, The Chef's soap, Desert Essence, Dr. Bronner's, Ecco Bella, and Tropical. Look for the words *vegetable oil–based soap* or *castile soap*.

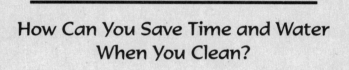

How Can You Save Time and Water When You Clean?

Here are my favorite cleaning tips. Even some professionals don't know them, but now you do. They will save you water and *time*, too!

1. ***Don't use too much cleaner.*** It's fun to squirt and spray, but if you put on too much, you make more work for yourself when it comes time to rinse. A well-designed cleaner and formula easily dispenses just the right amount for the job. Beware of containers that encourage you to overuse—most of them do.
2. ***Clean horizontal surfaces first.*** Horizontal surfaces collect the dirt. Don't waste time washing the clean vertical ones! Window sills; door frames; the top of the refrigerator; edges and tops of lamps, appliances, and TVs; shelves; mirror edges; and the tops of picture frames are all examples of the dirty and forgotten areas in your home.

3. *Work from top to bottom.* Going from top to bottom saves you water and time. *Check out the top of any room first before you start cleaning what's at eye level.* Cobwebs, window sills, and the tops of bookcases all cause problems if you clean them last. When I wipe a sill above a tub, sometimes a line of brown silt comes rolling down the tile walls. If I wait until I finish cleaning everything else to wipe that sill, then I have to rinse all over again. You get the picture.

4. *Wipe first, then rinse.* It's more fun to splash that water around, but save the fun for bathtime. If you monitor your water and time use closely, you will use a dry rag to wipe first and a wet sponge to rinse last. Use a vinegar rinse to dissolve a bit of the soap or baking-soda residue and you'll have to rinse even less.

5. *Use liquid soaps instead of liquid detergents.* Liquid detergents suds up well but can take five to 10 times more rinsing. Detergents leave a sticky film, too.

6. *Keep your cleaning items organized in a caddy or basket.* If you keep your cleaning basket stocked with fresh rags and cleaners, you'll save lots of time. Grab that basket and bring it to wherever and whatever you need cleaning and you're set. You should have everything you need—no running back and forth to get another cleaner or another rag. I have several cleaning baskets—one under the bathroom sink, one in the laundry room, and one in the garage. Even under the kitchen sink, a basket keeps things orderly and helps you to notice when you're missing something or running low. Make sure to get one with a sturdy handle.

7. *My favorite water-saving tip: keep a bucket in the tub!* Not all of you will like this suggestion, but some of you will. I keep a bucket in the tub when I take a shower. When I turn the sprayer on to heat the water up, the bucket catches all that otherwise wasted water. Afterward, I use the water in the bucket to

water my indoor and outdoor plants. But don't immediately water your plants with hot shower water; they won't like it. Let it cool down first. Bucket shower water makes great laundry water, too. If your shower is near the washer you can dump that water in the washer until the next wash. I know one family who swears by it. Keeping that bucket in the bathroom makes it handy for cleaning jobs, too. I have a nice powder-blue bucket and have gotten used to its presence in the tub. Thanks to my littlest sister for this great water-conservation tip.

Can You Really Let Your Kids Use These Cleaners?

With these alternative cleaners, you don't have to wait until your children take a nap to clean. Now with these cleaners you can spend their naptime doing something you enjoy. Clean with nontoxics while they're awake and teach them how to clean at the same time. I keep mine occupied with baby-type cleaning while I do the real stuff.

The cleaners to let your kids use are Club Clean™ glass cleaner and EarthShaker™ kitchen cleanser. You can let older ones use Momma's Earth Mop™ floor cleaner and

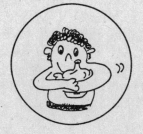

Earth Scrub™ tub and tile cleaner. Kids love to make baking soda fizz with a squirt-bottle of vinegar, but it's best to supervise it. Kids have a tendency to squirt each other in the eye with vinegar, and that can hurt. Using any liquid soap needs to be supervised, for similar reasons.

Following are some of the many ways I have cleaned with my child.

Everybody Wants to Clean!

One night, we had some neighborhood children over. They were acting kind of rowdy, so I decided to channel their energy into something positive. Okay, *what about cleaning?* I thought. The kids' ages ranged from 2 to 7 years. I got out a couple of spray-bottles, filled them with club soda, and introduced the concept. The spray-bottle was an immediate success, and all the children wanted their own. While I was getting out the rest of the spray-bottles, I started one of the kids cleaning a dusty toy on the porch and another wiping the mirrors. Soon, the house was silent. They were all busy, wiping and cleaning. I couldn't believe it. I decided to introduce the baking soda next. I grabbed a container of EarthShaker™ and gave it to the 3-year-old. He seemed to love that and started cleaning a stepstool with it. The 7-year-old spied the shaker and wanted one. Okay, but should I let him have it inside the house? Why not? It's just baking soda and easy to clean up with a little vinegar. He took the shaker and disappeared. The next thing I heard was "Okay, now let's go clean the toilet." And he tromped off with a littler one following. I wandered into the bathroom and complimented them all. "What a wonderful job you are doing." "Oh, I clean at my dad's house all the time." He seemed so proud. Cleaning is natural. Now that you have nontoxics, you can finally let your children help you clean.

BABY'S FIRST CLEANING EXPERIENCE

While I was carrying my daughter around in a front-style baby carrier, I used Club Clean™, my club-soda glass cleaner, to sparkle up my windows and mirrors. With the club soda, you don't have to worry about an ammonia smell around or chemical drips on that sensitive, sweet little baby. Most babies enjoy watching you squirt and wipe the window. It also makes the task of carrying around that baby a little less boring for you. As soon as my daughter was old enough to walk, I handed her a spray-bottle of club soda and showed her how to spray and wipe. She's been cleaning windows with her own little spray-bottle ever since.

BAKING SODA IN THE TUB

One day, I was cleaning around the tub with my baking-soda cleanser while my little one was taking a bath. She spied the pile of baking soda I had sprinkled on the side and started playing with it. Great. I told her it was soap. She loved it. After that, the baking soda thing became a bathtime ritual. "More soap," she'd say. I'd make her a little pile on the side of the tub and she would endlessly scoop it up, rinse her fingers, and watch it dissolve. Occasionally, she would taste a tiny bit of it and make a face. Since the doctor had told me to rub a little bit of baking soda on her teeth at night, I figured that a little baking soda in her mouth voluntarily was the most effortless tooth brushing I could ever get. She played while I cleaned.

WHISTLE WHILE YOU WORK

To teach your child how to clean, you've got to make it fun. For piles of spilled crayons, Legos, and assorted toys I use a song from Barney: "Clean up, clean up, everybody, everywhere. Clean up, clean up, everybody do your share." I start singing and cleaning, and my toddler inevitably comes over to help. I have even caught her spontaneously cleaning up her toys while singing this song. It's magic. Don't make spilling things bad; just make the cleaning up fun. As those toddlers get older, they will naturally lose interest in the fun of spilling (we hope).

However, be careful with sprayers. If you successfully teach your toddler to clean mirrors with Club Clean™, do so with this caution. Children should not be taught that they can use *any* spray-bottle—only the special bottles you say that they can use. Any areas where your children play without your supervision should not have spray-bottles with chemical products in them within reach. If you can't be assured of this, then don't teach your kids to use spray-bottles until they are old enough to know the difference. We want to solve problems with these alternative cleaners, not create new ones. I solved this problem by having a special small teal-colored sprayer with club soda in it that is baby's sprayer. That's "her" sprayer. All other sprayers are off limits. This caution holds for shakers and squirt containers, too. Teach children that they can use only the "kid kind" of cleaners.

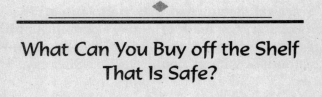

What Can You Buy off the Shelf That Is Safe?

Unfortunately, there are not very many products that I can suggest. Get the Washington Toxics Coalition's *Buy Smart, Buy Safe* guide and you will see a precise environmental rating of many name-brand cleaners (see Resources section, pp. 283–89). If you must buy off-the-shelf products, below is a list of my suggestions. I've included only name brands for your ease at the market. In some categories, there just wasn't a product that I could suggest in good conscience. This is not a comprehensive review or scientific rating of commercial cleaning products, just my personal suggestions from my own readings and experiences.

At the health-food store, I suggest all of the EarthRite or EarthWise products. At the supermarket, I'd get:

All-purpose sprays: **Planet** or **Cinch**
All-purpose cleaners for bathroom, kitchen, and floors: **Planet, Mr. Clean** (liquid), **Spic and Span** (liquid)
Bleach: **Clorox 2** all-fabric bleach (liquid)
Carpet spot removers: **Resolve** in the pump spray or **Woolite** spot and stain rug cleaner
Wood floor cleaners: **Murphy's Oil Soap**
Furniture polishes: **Lemon Pledge** (nonaerosol)
Glass cleaners: **Cinch** or **Planet**
Insecticides: Any trap or barriers without poisons, such as the popular, sticky **Roach Motel** or the tricky plastic yellow jacket traps
Kitchen cleansers: **Bon Ami**
Laundry stain removers: **Spray 'n Wash** stain stick
Toilet bowl cleaners: **Toilet Duck** or **Bon Ami** cleanser

---

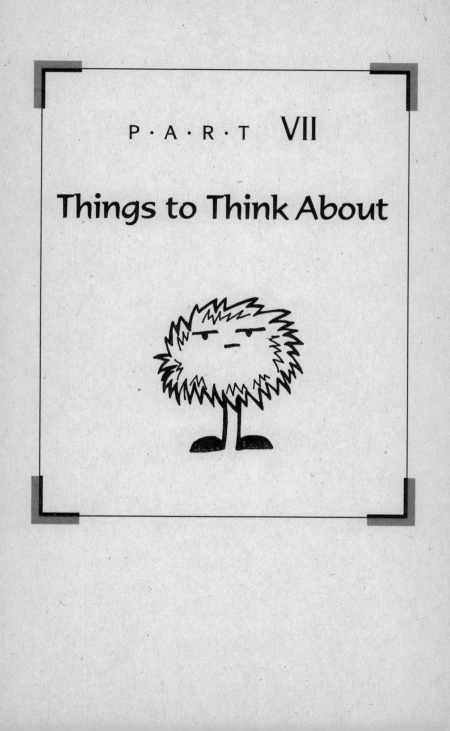

P·A·R·T **VII**

Things to Think About

What Is Nontoxic?

What do I mean when I call a cleaner nontoxic? It's really very simple. When I use the word *nontoxic* in this book, I don't mean it strictly technically, but as most people would understand it. Most people would consider ingredients such as baking soda, club soda, vinegar, salt, and lemon and lime juice to be nontoxic. But technically speaking, all of the above ingredients can be considered quite toxic. "The dose is the poison" is the often-quoted phrase. For example, if you eat enough salt, you can get very sick and even die. Some companies like to refer to their toxic products as "safe as salt," which of course then means that if you eat enough of it, you can get very sick and even die. Therefore, the chemical they are referring to as "safe as salt" might not be very safe at all for human use. It gets confusing when one person is talking about a technical definition and the other person is referring to the household meaning of the word.

Here's what I mean when I call a cleaner nontoxic:

- *Nontoxic cleaners are cleaners that you can use relatively safely, as compared to other commercial cleaning products (which range from fairly safe to extremely dangerous).* That also means that the cleaning ingredients are fairly nontoxic to humans to ingest, absorb, or breathe. For example, most of us would consider liquid soaps and hand-dishwashing detergents to be somewhat nontoxic, even though we realize that if we eat the soap, we can get sick and that we need to keep soap out of our eyes. Liquid soaps aren't scary to us because we know how to use them safely and what happens if we don't. *Saying that a cleaner is nontoxic doesn't mean that you can safely eat them, pour them all over your body, squirt them in your eyes, or do other crazy stuff.* But it can mean that if an accident should happen with them, such as a child's eating a little or your spilling a little, you or your child won't end up in the emergency room.

- *I've expanded the definition of* nontoxic *to include cleaners that are made out of ingredients that are fairly well understood.* New chemicals may be found out to be toxic in the future, and I don't think you should call a cleaner nontoxic unless you are pretty sure of your ingredients' track records.

- *I also think it is important to consider the toxicity of cleaners in the context of their ordinary use and disposal.* For example, if it's a cleaner that you use for washing the car and it's going to run down a storm drain and pollute a stream, then I try to suggest a soap that biodegrades as quickly as possible. *If it's a cleaner that is easy to inhale when using it and the bottle tells you not to breathe it, then I call it ridiculous and toxic!* Where, how, and when a cleaner is normally used and disposed of is the correct context in which to consider its degree of toxicity.

- To every definition, there are exceptions! In some of the recipes in this book, I have included borax, an ingredient that I consider to have some toxicity to humans and to the environment. But I have tried to make smart choices about where I've suggested that you use borax and how much to use.

But that's about it. Most people consider olive oil, baking soda, lemon juice, salt, club soda, and vinegar to be nontoxic ingredients. Most people agree that using snakes over chemical drain cleaners, pumice stones over acidic toilet bowl cleaners, and oven liners over fume-filled oven cleaners is better for everybody.

People seem to have a lot of trouble with the definition of *nontoxic*. I've heard quite a number of confusing arguments about it. The ordinary person wants nontoxic products but doesn't know what the word *nontoxic* really means; scientists have tried to define it technically but can't; cleaning companies have tried to define it to suit their needs; laws don't yet define it clearly; and finally, I've tried to define it by writing an entire book on it. Unfortunately, we all seem to define it quite differently.

We should all remember that for every word in the English language, there is a context. The majority of words that we learned as children were learned in context. How I use a particular word in a sentence helps to define its meaning. How we use particular words in society also creates their definitions. *Not very many people realize this, but the very definitions in our dictionaries change based on the way we decide to use our words.* Even this book interactively helps to define what the word *nontoxic* means. That's the wonderful thing about language: I can define *what I mean by* nontoxic *in the context of this book.* Marvelous.

What Makes These Cleaners Safer?

As you might imagine, the companies that sell cleaning products might not be thrilled about your making your own cleaning products at home for pennies. You might even expect some of them to launch a few advertising campaigns on the hazards of homemade products. Just in case things get that ridiculous, I've included a few points here for you to consider.

What makes my homemade recipes generally safer than the commercial products?

Safer Ingredients

No debate here. Ingredients like baking soda, liquid castile soap, and vinegar are milder and much safer to you and the environment as compared to ingredients like bleach, lye, and harsh acids such as sulfuric, phosphoric, and hydrofluoric acids. Generally speaking, I've substituted the full range of commercial cleaners with simple, safe homemade cleaners.

You might have a debate if you try to compare some of the safer commercial products with some of my recipes. In this case, consider using a milder commercial product if you like. (See p. 271 for a list of suggested commercial cleaners or get the *Buy Smart, Buy Safe Guide* [see Resources, p. 287].)

You Know All the Ingredients When You Make It Yourself

Commercial cleaning product labels are **not** *required to list all the ingredients*. That means you cannot make an educated choice about whether you want to purchase that product based on the ingredients. A company can include a poisonous or untested chemical and you won't even know. Even worse, your Poison Control Center also might have trouble finding out what's in it!

I've Tried to Give You Tools, Tips, and Cleaning Know-How in Place of Using Hazardous Chemicals

Using a harsh chemical to solve your cleaning problem may seem easier, but it can create hazards for you and the environment at the same time. Since the chemicals in oven cleaners, drain cleaners, and toilet bowl cleaners can be particularly hazardous, I've tried to encourage you to use mechanical methods, such as aluminum oven liners, plumbing snakes, and pumice stones, instead.

How do you know that these cleaning recipes are truly safer for the environment? I do *not* have a staff of 20 scientists who have spent the last 5 years testing my cleaning recipes against all the commercial equivalents for biodegradability, toxicity in disposal, or production. I do not need to because, practically speaking, baking soda, liquid castile soap, and vinegar are well known for their mildness to humans and the environment. Synthetic chemicals are not.

The only questionable ingredient I've included in my recipes is borax, and if you are a purist like me, you don't need to use it at all. I've included it in a few of my recipes because it bleaches mineral stains, helps to clean in harder water, and has reputed (but not proven) antifungal and antiseptic qualities.

◆

Calling Those 8oo Numbers

I've called a lot of 800 numbers that are listed on the backs of commercial cleaning product cans, bottles, and boxes; they are not all equal!

The prize for the most friendly, helpful, and informative goes to Arm & Hammer's excellent consumer line. The people you talk to are friendly, intelligent, and full of clear instructions about how and what you can use baking soda for. Take advantage of this excellent service and find out more about this miracle mineral.

The prize for the rudest consumer hotline goes to Procter & Gamble,* the company that makes a truckful of cleaning products like Tide, Palmolive, Cascade, and Mr. Clean. I consistently got robotlike people on the phone who sounded like they were reading back to me a two- or three-line message appearing on their computer screen regarding a particular product or question. They consistently became very disturbed and angry if I wanted any more information. They would repeat their dogmatic message again and then say that they just didn't know anything beyond that. Quite frustrating, to say the least.

The award for the absolutely worst hotline goes to Reckitt & Colman, which makes products such as Black Flag insecticides, Easy-Off oven cleaners, and Red Devil drain opener. This company doesn't even *have* a consumer hotline on some of their products' labels. Without a consumer hotline, you have no way to easily get information on the product or voice complaints. Even the all-important medical emergency number can be small and hard to find on their labels. When I called their medical emergency line, the person who answered the phone would not give out even the most basic information on the hazards of the product.

---

*P&G is a huge, global economic force netting over $4 billion in sales a year. You can hardly avoid buying at least one of their products on every shopping trip. A company as big as this has a huge environmental impact. Let them know that you demand that they be environmentally responsible. It's easy to call their 800 line. The packaging from their products alone accounts for over 1% of the total garbage in the United States. P&G is in a great position to help reduce our waste problem but has reportedly lobbied against legislation regarding the problem, although they have voluntarily started several noteworthy programs to reduce packaging themselves. As a consumer, you are in the driver's seat with your little wad of grocery money. Companies listen to customers.

Dear Reader . . .

I hope you have enjoyed reading about these nontoxic recipes. This book is my hope for the planet. Now, it's up to you. You've been trained to clean differently, so the hardest part will be getting into the habit of making your cleaners yourself. You may think it's a hassle and it's going to take too much time. It's not, and it isn't. But you need to try it, because you won't believe me until you see for yourself. Get the essential oils, make up a couple of gallons of scented vinegar and three or four boxes of scented baking soda, and you will naturally start using them. Having the containers with the recipes on the labels helps. You might even find the person in your family who "never cleans" making up a recipe or two. This nontoxic cleaning thing is a simple solution to a complex, expensive, and environmentally damaging problem. *You* make the difference. Please let me know what's working and what's not. I'm always looking for better recipes. Call or write. I'd love to hear from you.

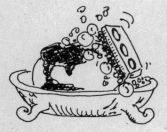

Karen Logan
Life on the Planet
23852 Pacific Coast Hwy #200
Malibu, CA 90265
(818) 880-5144

RESOURCES

◆

Bottles and Containers

Where to get cleaning bottles and containers with the recipes right on the labels? From my company, Life on the Planet, of course!

Life on the Planet
23852 Pacific Coast Hwy #200
Malibu, CA 90265
(818) 880-5144
Fax: (818) 880-5417
On the Internet: http://www.cleanhouse.com

Life on the Planet is dedicated to earth-friendly, non-toxic cleaning products for everyone, everywhere. We offer unfilled (yes, empty!) bottles and containers with the nontoxic recipes right on the labels. We also offer a set of printed recipe labels, alone, and laminated recipe cards. Call us up and ask us about any cleaning question you desire or tell us about a nontoxic cleaning tip you've discovered.

Essential Oils

Frontier Herbs (catalog company)
2264 Market Street
San Francisco, CA 94114
(800) 786-1388
(415) 621-8444

This is a cooperative company with thousands of products. Enjoy looking in their catalog but don't get lost. For cleaning, all you need is a few essential oils. I suggest the ⅓-oz. bottles of peppermint, lemon, lavender, and tea tree oils. They also offer certified organic essential oils. While organic is more expensive, if you buy organic, you will still save a significant amount of money by making your own cleaning products. Go for it.

Liquid Soap Companies

All-One-God-Faith
Rabbi Dr. E. H. Bronner Associates, SMMC
P.O. Box 28
Escondido, CA 92033
(619) 747-2211

Dr. Bronner's liquid castile soaps come in peppermint, almond, lavender, eucalyptus, and unscented in the following sizes: 4, 8, 16, and 32 oz.; ½ gallon, and 1 gallon. They also sell very high quality peppermint and lavender oils.

If you don't have a health-food store nearby, you can order Dr. Bronner's soaps from The Magic Chain at (800) 622-6648.

Desert Essence
9510 Vassar Avenue, Unit A
Chatsworth, CA 91311
(818) 709-8525
(800) 709-5900

You can get tea tree oil and tea tree oil liquid soap from this environmentally conscious company. I had the good fortune to meet the man who brought wonderful tea tree oil to America and the founder of the Desert Essence, Steven Silberfein. He has developed over 100 excellent products with tea tree oil in them for you to enjoy.

Cleaning Companies and Catalogs

Don Aslett's Cleaning Center (catalog company)
P.O. Box 39
311 South 5th Avenue
Pocatello, ID 83204
(800) 451-2402

Don Aslett's a funny guy with funny cleaning books that are full of very practical tips. His cleaners are not even close to being chemical-free, but his practical know-how is worth its weight in gold. Products you might consider getting are the Maid's Basket, Don's Famous Cleaning Cloths (utility cloths), the Ettore window squeegee, grout brush, shower squeegee with hook to hang in the shower, and carpet mats.

The Clean Team (catalog company)
2264 Market Street
San Francisco, CA 94114
(415) 621-8444

The Clean Team is a fabulous cleaning service available in the San Francisco Bay Area started by Jeff Campbell, author of *Speed Cleaning*. He also has a catalog that you can get by calling (800) 717-CLEAN. You will find lots of useful, professional cleaning tools and supplies here. I'd consider getting the whisk broom, professional toothbrush, and window and shower squeegees. For your heavy-duty cleaning tools, consider getting a heavy-duty scraper, razor-blade holder, tile brush, and pumice stone. The scraper and the razor-blade holder are less expensive if you get them from a hardware store. For my house, I almost never use heavy-duty cleaning tools but they are great to have when you need them. It's better to be prepared with tools than to have to resort to harsh chemicals. Don't be tempted to get the cleaning apron as I did. I never used it. It's great if you are a professional and you are going to clean a big house for several hours. I almost never clean like that. I usually clean in bits and pieces, grabbing things conveniently from under the counters or carrying them to where I need them in a basket or caddie.

Ecoproducts Catalog Companies

Seventh Generation (catalog company)
49 Hercules Drive
Colchester, VT 05446
(800) 456-1177

Seventh Generation has a great catalog for environmentally responsible stuff. If you want to try some of the premade ecocleaning products, this is a good place to start. They also have lots of other ecohome items. I suggest a composting bin and bucket or bags, energy-saving fluorescent lightbulbs, rechargeable battery unit (get the unit that handles all sizes; it's worth it), terry cotton–covered mop, carpet sweeper (they have a better price than the one from The Clean Team), and anything made with organic cotton. Treat yourself to some organic cotton sheets if you can afford it. I have some, and they are delicious to sleep in; they're pretty, soft, sweet smelling, and environmentally kind.

Real Goods (catalog company)
555 Leslie Street
Ukiah, CA 95482
(800) 762-7325

The people at Real Goods are the national experts and pioneers of energy-saving environmentally designed homes—great catalog, great company. They are the company to go to when you're ready to get serious about solar energy. If you are not ready for that, you can enjoy their other resource-saving products. I suggest starting with the green plug (saves energy on your refrigerator), solar-powered rechargeable battery unit and other gadgets, low-flow shower heads and nozzles, smart mousetrap, and window insulators. Their books and workshops are gold mines of information and experience in ecoproducts and living.

Environmental Organizations

Washington Toxics Coalition
4516 University Way NE
Seattle, WA 98105
(206) 632-1545

This environmental organization is producing outstanding research and publications on the toxicity of commercial products and their least-toxic alternatives. Philip Dickey, the master scientist there, has a doctoral degree in nuclear physics. His approach is rational, in-depth, intelligent, and determined. Get his most recent publication, called *Buy Smart, Buy Safe*. In it, he reviews the toxicity and environmental impact of both "green" commercial cleaning products and the brand-name cleaners you'll find in your supermarket. His findings are sometimes quite surprising.

Government Organizations

Debbie Raphael
Environmental Program Division, City of Santa Monica
200 Santa Monica Pier, Suite F
Santa Monica, CA 90401
(310) 458-2213

Santa Monica is the most environmentally hip city that I know of (okay, Seattle comes to mind as well). Santa Monica is consistently doing boundary-breaking things. Most recently, they drew up a program to require that all the cleaners that the city uses be as environmentally safe as possible. The program was really implemented, and it really worked. The janitors actually use the safer cleaners. If your city wants to know how they did it, call them up. They are terrific and very friendly.

Pest Control

Bio-Integral Resource Center (BIRC)
P.O. Box 7414
Berkeley, CA 94707
(510) 524-2567

This center has the national experts on least-toxic pest control. Write or call them for practical, tried-and-true answers to your pest problems. They provide this valuable information to you for free, so support them by getting a membership, buying a book, or purchasing one of their many publications. Organizations like BIRC are paving the way to least-toxic pest controls for industry and home use. It's an important contribution to the health and well-being of the planet. Support it.

National Coalition Against the Misuse of Pesticides
(NCAMP)
701 E Street SE
Washington, D.C. 20003
(202) 543-5450

This is another great environmental organization dedicated to public health and alternatives to pesticides.

ACKNOWLEDGMENTS

◆

Thanks to:

Mark, for his advice, endless support, and love.

Sophie, my 2-year-old, for contributing numerous cleaning opportunities for testing my recipes.

Keith, for his belief in the project, love for the planet, and inspiration.

Bonnie, for her creativity, dedicated work, and practical wisdom.

Patagonia, for the initial funding of an environmental idea out of which this book eventually grew.

Tess and Pam at Earth Angels, for my first wholesale order of products and for introducing me to my agent, Charlotte.

Ally Sheedy, for appreciating my products and getting her mom involved.

Charlotte Sheedy, my agent, for getting me a great book contract.

Emily Bestler, my editor, for loving the products, appreciating my ideas, and bringing this book to you.

INDEX

LIFE ON THE PLANET TO YOU

◆

My company is all about making it easy for you to use these nontoxic cleaning recipes. Getting the right container and having the recipe right on the label makes these homemade cleaners easy and fun. I don't fill the bottles for you because I don't like the idea of paying to ship you mostly water. It might be nice to have the first bottle filled for you because it's your habit to buy a bottle off the shelf, use its contents up, and throw it away, but if I send you an empty bottle, you can get off to the right start by making the cleaners and filling it yourself.

I keep my prices on the containers as affordable as possible, but because we are a small company, we don't get the huge volume discounts (yet?) to pass on to you. You can also buy a set of recipe labels separately that you can put on your own containers. I've tried to include all the information that you will need on every label.

I'd love to hear from you. If you send me a self-addressed, stamped envelope, I will send you a *free* reference card with the best of my recipes on it. Having a reference card makes refilling your bottles easy. When you get it, tape it to the inside of one of your kitchen cupboards, and you will always be able to find it when you need it.

Happy cleaning!

Karen Logan
Life on the Planet
23852 Pacific Coast Hwy #200
Malibu, CA 90265(818)
880-5144
Fax: (818) 880-5417

Life on the Planet